Fit**KIDS**

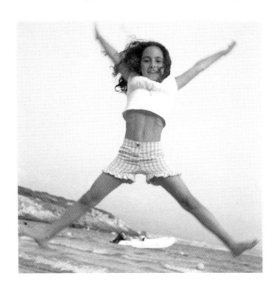

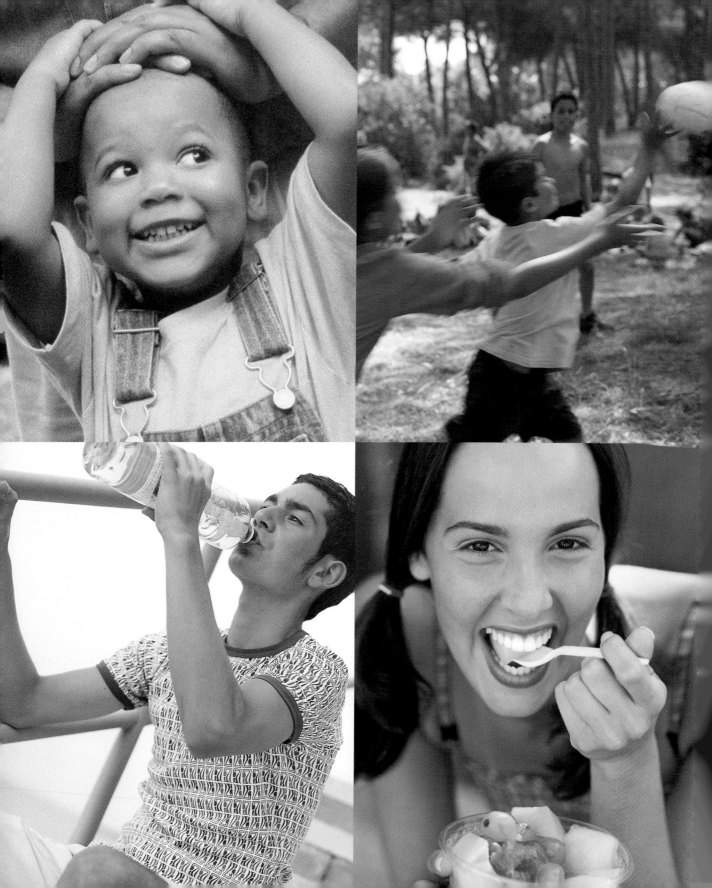

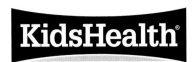

Fit KIDS

A practical guide to raising active and healthy children – from birth to teens

Mary L. Gavin MD
Steven A. Dowshen MD
Neil Izenberg MD

Foreword by
Dr Jane Collins
Chief Executive, Great Ormond Street Hospital for Sick Children

LONDON, NEW YORK, MUNICH, MELBOURNE, DELHI

Project Editor Norma MacMillan

Senior Managing Editor Jemima Dunne

Design XAB Design

DTP Designer Julian Dams

Managing Art Editor Marianne Markham

Production Controller Louise Daly

Category Publishers Mary Thompson, Corinne Roberts

Art Director Bryn Walls

Nutritionist for UK edition Fiona Hunter BSc Hons (Nutri.), Dip. Dietetics

KIDSHEALTH

Editor Debra Moffitt

Medical Editors Sandra G. Hassink MD, Jessica Donze RD, MPH

Consulting Chef Niklaus Fuster

This edition first published in United Kingdom in 2004 by Dorling Kindersley Limited
80 Strand, London, WC2R 0RL
A Penguin Company

Fit Kids provides information on a wide range of health and medical topics.
The book is not a substitute for medical diagnosis, however, and you are advised always to consult your doctor for
specific information on personal health matters.

Any recipes in this book are intended for people of generally good health, without specific food allergies.

A CIP record for this book is available from the British Library
ISBN 1 4053 047 66

Colour reproduction by Colourscan, Singapore
Printed and bound in Singapore by Star Standard Industries (Pte.) Ltd.

Foreword

The good news for parents is that most children nowadays are healthier than those of any other generation. Serious or even fatal illnesses, in particular those due to infections, are now either preventable or treatable. Unfortunately, though, a new problem faces parents today: childhood obesity, which was relatively rare even one or two decades ago, is becoming a major problem in the UK, as it is in all other developed countries. More than a third of British children are now overweight. There were overweight children before, but the number is increasing rapidly year on year. It is something we should all be concerned about.

Being overweight is a problem for a child. It often causes low self-esteem and therefore lack of confidence, as well as health problems such as musculo-skeletal and respiratory problems and even a form of diabetes that was previously only seen in adults. An overweight child has a high risk of being an overweight adult. Long-term health consequences include hypertension, heart disease, diabetes, musculo-skeletal problems, and an increased risk of a number of common cancers.

As a parent it can sometimes be difficult to acknowledge that your child is becoming overweight.

It is much easier to recognize it in your friends' children or when you see children out and about. If parents do start to think about it in their own child they often aren't sure what to do. Many parents say to me that they are worried about mentioning weight to their child, particularly to a daughter, in case it precipitates an eating disorder.

Fit Kids has been written by experts to help you prevent your child from becoming overweight and to help you if he or she already is. It describes what you can do to develop healthy eating patterns and keep your children fit. It does this in a realistic way, recognizing the pressures of our modern-day lives. I hope this book will help your children to grow up fit and healthy.

Jane Colli

Dr Jane Collins
Chief Executive, Great Ormond Street
Hospital for Sick Children

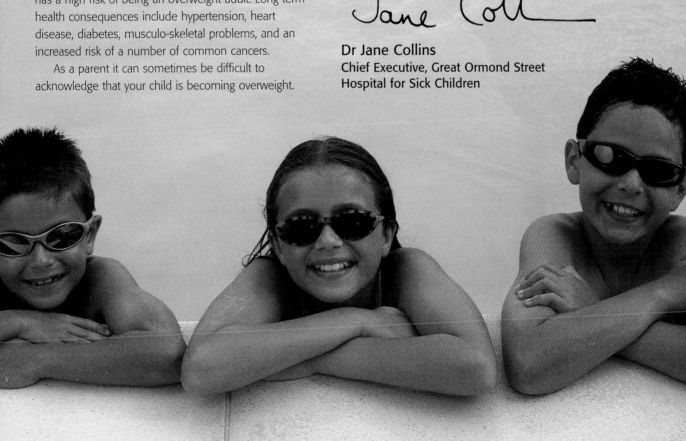

Contents

Introduction   8

1 Children's weight and fitness   10
Healthy for life   12
Look at your child's development   16
Overweight children   20
Take a family approach   24

2 Principles of nutrition   30
The vital components of food   32
A healthy diet for children   40
How to help kids eat healthier   44
Be an informed food shopper   46

3 Principles of fitness   50
Fit and healthy for life   52
How to get physically fit   56
Playing safe   64

4 The first year   68
Making a good start   70
Nutrition in the first year of life   72
Activity for babies   84

5 Toddlers: 1–3 years   92
Toddlers on the move   94
Nutrition for toddlers   96
Activity for toddlers   104

6 Pre-school kids: 3–5 years   108
Taking their place in the world   110
Nutrition for pre-school kids   112
Activity for pre-school kids   118

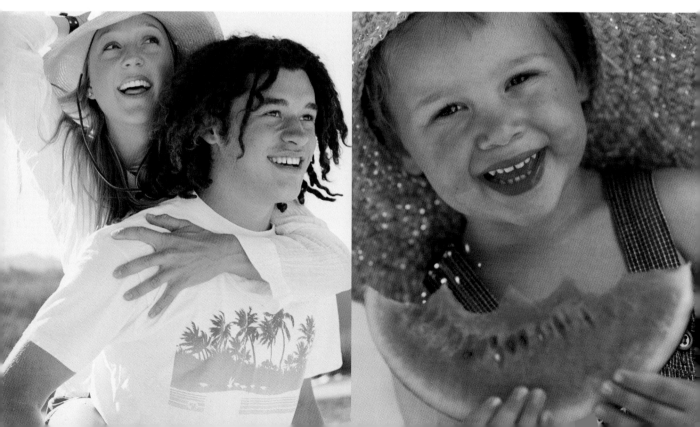

7 School-age kids: 6–12 years — 122

A time of dramatic change — 124
Nutrition for school-age kids — 126
Fitness for school-age kids — 136
Puberty in school-age children — 146

8 Adolescents: 13–18 years — 148

Becoming mature — 150
Nutrition for teenagers — 152
Fitness for teenagers — 164

9 Special concerns — 170

Special challenges — 172
The child with food allergies — 174
The child with diabetes — 176
Helping all children be active — 178
The child with special needs — 180
The child athlete — 182

10 Healthy recipes — 186

Good food for good health — 189
Breakfasts to start the day — 191
Take time for lunch — 192
Sit down to dinner — 196
Snacks and smoothies — 200

Recommended resources — 202

Index — 204

Acknowledgments — 208

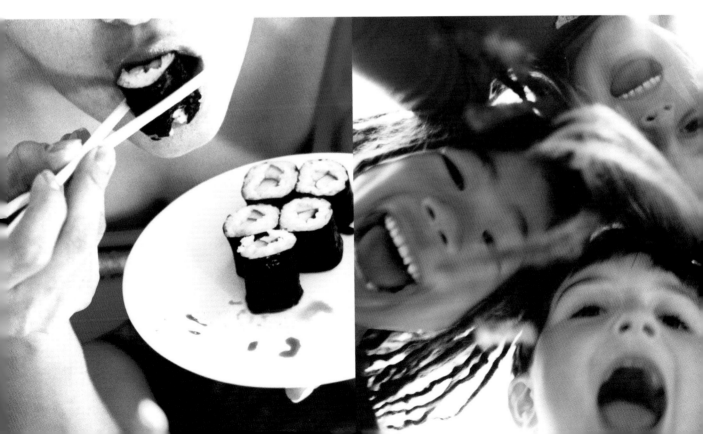

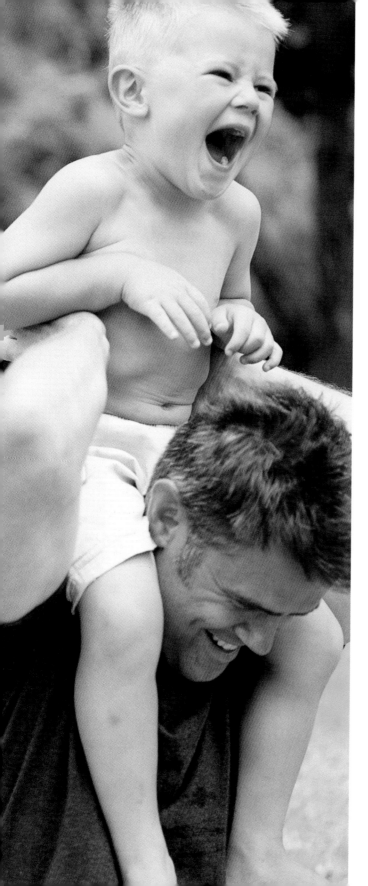

Introduction

We're living longer than any time in history. Children born today in this country have every hope of living to their 80s, 90s – or even beyond. The quality and availability of health care has improved dramatically in the last few decades. We now have year-round access to better, more plentiful foods than ever before. We know more about vitamins and nutrition, and that – amazingly – a proper diet can ward off serious medical conditions, including certain cancers, heart disease, and diabetes. More than ever, we value exercise, respect both women's and men's athletics, and acknowledge the importance of maintaining lifelong fitness.

So our children (and we parents) should be in the greatest physical shape ever, shouldn't we? Well…not exactly. It's true for some of us. But many parents and children are struggling. Despite the proliferation of slimming foods, diet plans, and gyms, we're not in the shape we want to be. In fact, we could do a lot better.

More and more people are overweight

We are fatter than we were even a generation ago – and the rate of obesity is rising alarmingly. Seats in theatres and cinemas and on buses will need to be redesigned to accommodate our widening seats. But squeezing into our seats (or our trousers) isn't the worst part. Our health – and the health of our kids – is at risk. Being overweight or out of shape also causes social and emotional pain, and often in a serious way.

The problem is that food tastes great. Our exquisitely sensitive tastebuds let us revel in the pleasures of rich chocolate ice cream and crispy chips. Our fridges and storecupboards are usually well stocked. Supermarket shelves groan under unlimited choices, and packaged foods are brilliantly engineered to appeal to our eyes and our palates. Food tempts us everywhere – at home, in our work places, and in our schools. Who can resist? Even petrol stations have become fast food markets, where you can grab a big bag of crisps, a pie, and an ultra-large sugary drink. It may be second nature to slurp and munch on the go, but it really adds up. Exceed your calorie needs by just an extra can of cola and a packet of crisps a day and you'll gain 12kg (26lb) in a year. You know what that means – another notch on your belt.

Food is not just fuel

It would be easier to resist if food were just about nutrition and getting "fuel" in our tanks. But food often means love, celebration, and family togetherness. Parents and grandparents have long rewarded children with food. And whether we're kids or adults, the process of eating feels good, even when we're not hungry. Food can easily become a consolation when we're feeling lonely or down. We deserve a little treat (or two), don't we?

We can't blame food alone. Our expanding waistlines have as much to do with our output (activity) as our input (eating). Most of us aren't active enough and there are good excuses: too little time and a lethargic lifestyle built around sedentary activities. It's easy to sit at a work desk all day and watch TV all night. Yet being physically active is the key to good health.

Children mimic their parents

Kids learn from their parents' patterns and imitate us, so why not set the kind of example you know they need? Maybe you were never good at sport and rarely exercise. Some children are the same way and may not enjoy organized team sports. But that doesn't mean you and your children can't be active, have fun, and stay in shape. You can do it without clocking long hours in the gym or enduring a lot of sweat and pain.

With food, too, you can set the right example. Make healthy eating a fun and delicious way of life, steering your children in the right direction, even as their needs change through the years. The aim is not to build elite athletes, or to put children on a fast cure-all diet. It's about getting children – all sorts of children – to adopt the lifelong habit of eating healthily and being active.

There is no quick fix

If anyone tells you that it's easy to get a child to eat well and stay active, they're kidding you. But there's reason to invest the effort now. Many adult health problems start in childhood – though they may not be recognized until much later, when it's harder to undo them. We want today's children to avoid those problems, so they can enjoy many years of fun, activity, and good health.

As paediatricians and health educators, we feel for families trying to adopt healthy habits and fight the threat of overweight. We also celebrate (though not with a slice of cake) the successes of many who are already walking the walk. With reasonable effort, thoughtfulness, and some planning, you can make nutrition and exercise a natural part of your family's life. What you'll get in return will be priceless: fit and healthy kids.

Neil Izenberg MD
Editor-in-Chief, KidsHealth

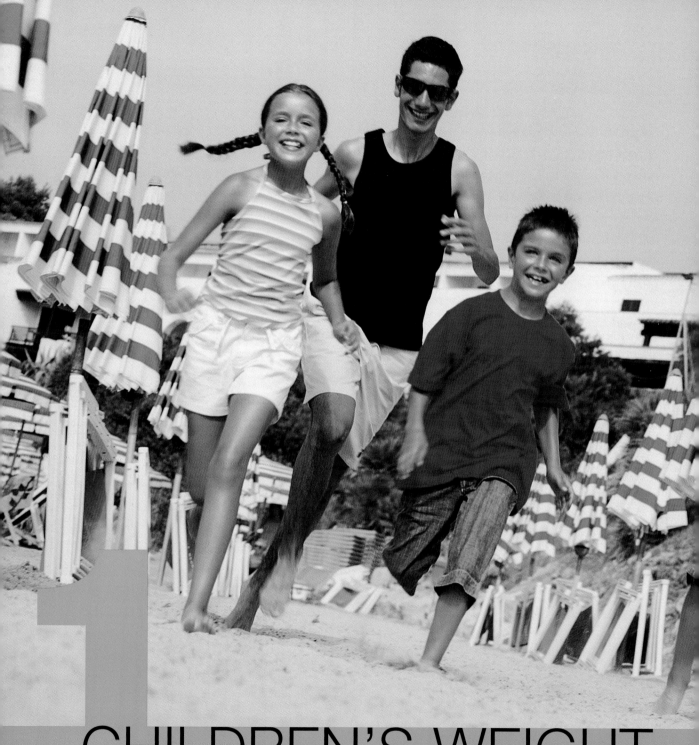

1 CHILDREN'S WEIGHT
AND FITNESS

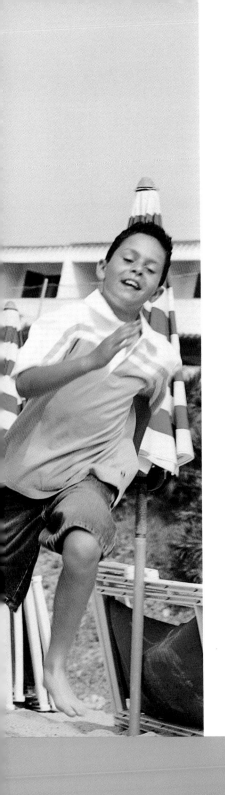

Eat right and be active – good advice that can be difficult to put into practice. But **you can help your children** do just that by setting a healthy table as well as **getting the whole family involved** in physical activity.

Healthy for life

It's a challenge to instil good eating and fitness habits in your children, which you'll know if you've ever substituted carrot sticks for crisps as snacks or tried to ration computer time.

Creating the foundation

You want the best for your children, especially when it comes to their health and well-being. You know how important food and fitness are for good health, as study after study has shown. And, as parents, you realize that making decisions about exercise and nutrition is a weighty responsibility. Children need nutritious food and physical activity for optimal growth and development, so how can you encourage healthy

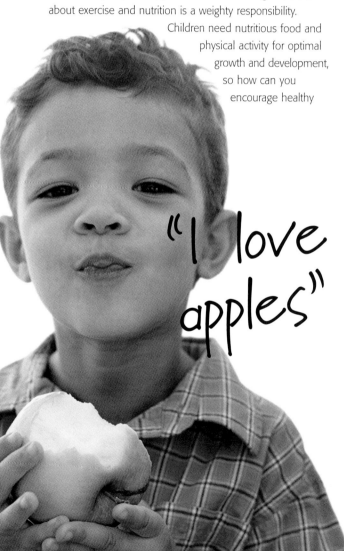

"I love apples"

habits in your family? If you aren't sure, you're not alone. As with all aspects of parenting, the aim is to create a foundation that will enable your children to make wise choices as they grow more independent.

The wrong signals

Some common strategies related to food, such as bribing children with dessert or making them eat everything on their plates, are easy options, but they send the wrong messages. They convey two incorrect ideas:

- Sweets are a reward.
- Hunger – or lack of it – has no bearing on the decision to keep eating or put down the fork.

A parent's attempts to get a child to exercise can backfire as well. For example, starting a child in team sports too young, or in a sport or activity that is beyond his or her ability, can lead to frustration and loss of interest.

Setting good examples

The family's daily habits and how parents live their own lives form a part of the child's landscape – what will be regarded as normal. Over time, the child will grow accustomed to the kinds of breakfast cereals that are in the cupboard, for example, and how Saturday mornings are spent, be it sleeping in or working out. No mum or dad will be perfect, but by making more good decisions than poor ones, parents can create an environment that supports the growth of a fit and healthy child.

This is by no means easy to do. Habits are ingrained and food is abundant. Modern lifestyles encourage eating on the move, as well as spending long hours sitting in cars, at computers, and in front of TVs. It can be hard to swim against this tide, but there are compelling reasons to do so: the number of overweight children – and adults – has risen dramatically and this trend upwards shows no sign of stopping. Making changes in the way your family operates can be a lifelong gift you give to your children.

Assessing your child's health

If you want to improve your child's health and well-being, it can be difficult to know where to begin. Here's some useful advice about assessing how things stand right now. It will also be useful as you continue to monitor how nutritious your child's eating habits are and his or her fitness levels throughout childhood.

Look at eating habits

Answer "yes" or "no" to these statements to determine how healthy your child's eating habits are:

- My child eats fruit every day.
- My child eats vegetables every day.
- My child eats a variety of foods, including dairy, whole grains, fruits, vegetables, and healthy sources of protein.
- My child usually eats only when hungry, not to relieve stress or boredom.
- My child will try new foods.
- Our family rarely eats meals or snacks in front of the TV.
- Our family eats together at least five times a week.

Look at exercise habits

Answer "yes" or "no" to these statements to determine how active your child is:

- My child gets physical activity every day.
- My child seems to enjoy being active.
- My child likes his or her body.
- Our family exercises together, such as taking walks, swimming, playing tag, or working in the garden.
- I make time to exercise on my own.
- I know how much physical activity is right for my child's age group.
- My child's favourite pastimes are active ones, such as sport, playing freely, or cycling.
- My child has access at home to a variety of sports and activity equipment, such as balls, bicycles, skipping ropes, and trainers.

What were your answers?

If you answered "yes" to a statement, you and your family have already adopted that healthy habit. If you answered "no", you are now able to identify what you need to do to make improvements in your family's lifestyle. Tackle the areas one at a time, if necessary, and work on them until you can say "yes" to all the statements.

Some areas may be more of a struggle than others or may grow in complexity as your son or daughter gets older. Also remember that you are an integral part of the picture. It might be illuminating to ask yourself the same assessment questions. Do you eat fruit every day, enjoy being active, and like your body? If you come up short, resolve that you and your child will start making progress together.

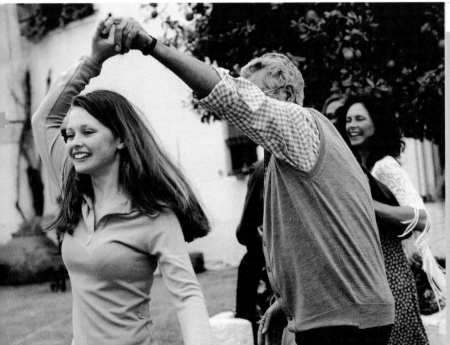

What parents say...
about being a role model

"We are a very close family – three generations – and do lots of things together. My parents, now in their 70s, are extremely active. They cycle and ramble, and enjoy square dancing, which my daughter also loves. My mum always cooked from scratch, and I follow her example with my own family. I try to set good examples for my kids with exercise too. I jog and do aerobics and weight-training, and as a family we do some kind of physical activity at the weekend."

21st-century challenges

With our modern lifestyles, it can be difficult to strike a healthy balance between calories consumed and energy expended through physical activity and exercise. There are many challenges for both parents and children.

Obstacles to overcome

Today, life has a one-two-three punch for anyone trying to maintain a healthy weight and lifestyle:

- a plentiful supply of food that's quick to buy or make and easy to overeat;
- sedentary routines, including long commutes, desk jobs, and free time spent in front of the TV or computer;
- daily schedules so jam-packed that it's difficult to find time to prepare wholesome family meals or exercise.

Even the most motivated parents, who take time to prepare a home-cooked meal, may find that their kids would rather eat a biscuit than a carrot, even with a delicious hummus dip. And they may resist trying new, healthy foods. Finding time for exercise also may seem impossible for working parents, especially if both of them work, as weekends are spent doing laundry and food shopping, not walking or playing cricket in the park. While parents try to tackle the household tasks, many kids may simply park themselves in front of the TV or computer, instead of being active.

Fast food

After long days at school and work, everyone is hungry. Yet many families are too worn out to wait for a healthy meal to be prepared and then to sit down to eat it together. As a result, convenience foods, which may be low in nutrients and high in fat, are staples in many households. And, of course, fast food is in plentiful supply.

It's not just what kids are eating: it's how much. The American trend of serving large portions as standard is becoming increasingly common in the UK. According to the National Obesity Forum, over the past decade portion sizes of fast foods and take-aways have increased by 30 percent.

Fast food portion sizes **on the rise**

In the last decade the portion size of many fast food items and manufactured foods has increased dramatically, resulting in mega servings of calories, fat, salt, and sugar. While a modest portion was once standard fare, many manufacturers and retailers are now offering "supersize" and "value meals" to tempt consumers to eat more. It's not uncommon these days to find restaurants offering "eat-as-much-as-you-can" dishes or for retailers to offer "meal deals" in which chips or a packet of crisps and a drink are included in with the price of a sandwich.

SUPERSIZED FAST FOOD IN THE US AND UK

FAST FOOD	US SIZE IN 1955	US SUPERSIZE IN 2002	UK SUPERSIZE IN 2003
Cola	200ml (7floz)	1.2l (42floz)	750ml (25.3floz)
Burger	45g (1.6oz)	225g (8oz)	215g (7.6oz)
Fries	70g (2.4oz)	201g (7.1oz)	185g (6.6oz)

INCREASED CALORIES, FAT, AND SUGAR

FAST FOOD	US SIZE IN 1955	US SUPERSIZE IN 2002	UK SUPERSIZE IN 2003
Fries	210 calories / 10g fat	610 calories / 29g fat	486 calories / 21g fat
Cola	85 calories / 24g sugar	500 calories / 140g sugar	323 calories / 79g sugar

Empty-calorie drinks

High consumption of sugary, calorie-dense drinks also contributes to weight gain among kids. Adolescents are drinking more cola, replacing healthier drinks such as milk, water, and 100-percent fruit juice. A survey by the National Dairy Council found that 60 percent of children consumed at least one fizzy drink a day and 22 percent had four or more each day. It's not just colas: many juice drinks and squashes are heavily sweetened. And, although it contains more nutrients, the calories from 100-percent juice can add up quickly if consumed in large quantities.

Drinking cola not only adds empty calories, it often goes hand in hand with snacking on high-calorie, high-fat foods. Cola is paired with fast food and other salty snacks, so it's natural for kids to associate the two. When they're drinking a cola, kids are more likely to reach for crisps than a piece of fresh fruit or vegetable. And, as it is, they're already not getting enough fruits and vegetables (see page 43).

A sedentary lifestyle

Before the conveniences of modern life – cars, washing machines, microwaves, televisions, computers, and so on – families spent more active time together doing household tasks, walking to school and work, and playing outdoors. But today daily life requires little physical activity.

As television viewing has increased, time spent in active work or play has decreased. Also many children snack in front of the TV, and research has shown a clear link between watching TV and being overweight. Many children can't, or aren't allowed to, walk or bike to school. And suburban neighbourhoods are often disconnected from the functional parts of towns, where a child could once have walked on his or her own to the library or a corner shop.

Even children who have physical education classes at school and participate in team sports may not be getting enough exercise. Currently in the UK, almost half of seven- to 11-year-olds get less than two hours of PE or school sport a week, which is the government target to be reached by 2006. As children get older, they're even less likely to be physically active. Changing that trend will mean changing the way parents and children think about sports and activity.

Parents may overlook the value of free play, especially for pre-adolescent children. But simply letting a child do his or her own thing may be a welcome break from lessons and sports practice. It also may result in more sustained activity.

Exercise is for everybody, not just the natural athletes among us. Later in the book, we'll talk about the value of an active lifestyle and introduce the concept of a "lifetime sport", which your child can enjoy for decades to come.

Time bind

Lengthy commutes, long work hours, and overscheduling leave little spare time for parents. Meanwhile, they are getting up earlier in the morning in an attempt to accomplish even more before the sun rises on the day.

Modern families feel so crunched by the demands of jobs, children's activities, and running the household that, more often than not, they don't eat meals together. For some families, eating at the family table happens only at birthdays and Christmas. That is unfortunate because a meal shared by the whole family is more likely to be nutritious. And it gives parents a chance to introduce children to new foods, to act as role models for healthy eating, and to talk.

Computer games can take over
Children younger than eight often spend two or more hours a day watching TV or playing computer games, while kids older than eight can spend four or more hours doing the same. Two hours maximum each day is a good guideline for all ages.

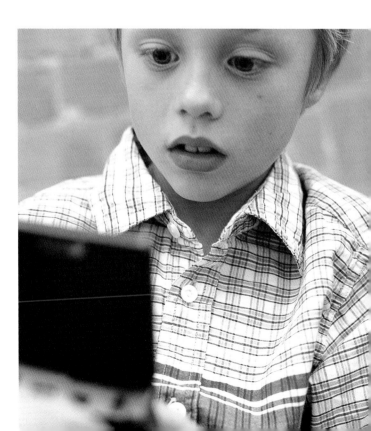

Look at your child's development

Growth is one of the most important indicators of a child's health. But remember that children come in many sizes and shapes and there's no one perfect weight or ideal body type.

Is my child growing properly?

Normal children develop at different rates, so even kids the same age as your child may be bigger or smaller, or at a different stage of physical maturity. In the early years, your child will be weighed and measured during regular check-ups with your GP. The readings can be plotted on a growth chart (see opposite) to follow your child's height and weight over time. You can plot your own chart at home too.

Understanding growth charts

From the moment your child is born, the measurements start, with your GP and health visitor documenting growth at each regular health review. Typically, infants are seen every few weeks by the health visitor, and by the GP at six to eight weeks, then at six to nine months and 18–24 months. The next check up is normally at around four years of age.

The curved lines on a growth chart represent percentiles. A percentile is based on a scale of 100. If your child is in the 50th percentile, half the children the same age are bigger and half are the same size or smaller.

On a growth chart, the lines indicate expected patterns of weight gain and height growth. It's ideal when height and weight percentiles are about the same, but they may differ depending on your child's build. Your child may be growing along a high, low, or middle percentile. It's not like a grade on a test – the 95th percentile is not better than the 50th. There can be some variation, but growth usually progresses along the same percentile. What you need to watch out for are sudden and major changes.

"I want to be this tall!"

Assessing **height and weight**

Parents in the UK are supplied with a Health Book in which they can plot their child's development. Height and weight are plotted on standardized charts (see page 208 for information about these). Charts make checking growth easy because you can see, at a glance, when a child who had been growing steadily veers off course. A single point on the chart provides a snapshot of how one child compares with other children who are the same age. But plotting your child's height and weight over time yields the most important information. This visual aid can offer reassurance that your child is growing properly or spot trends that need attention.

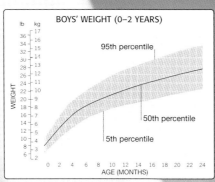

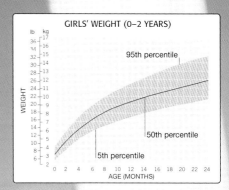

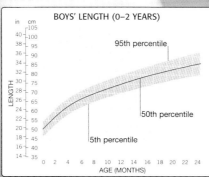

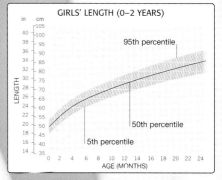

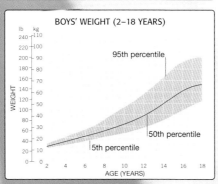

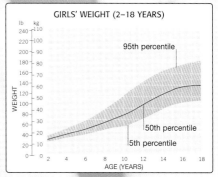

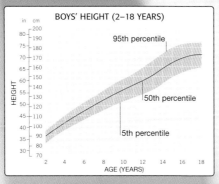

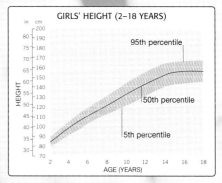

Is your child a healthy weight?

Although growth charts can be useful, Body Mass Index (BMI) charts are better for determining if a child is at a healthy weight. Using a formula, you can calculate your child's BMI and your GP can help you to interpret the results.

BMI and what it means

This is a way of using height and weight measurements to estimate how much body fat a person has. After calculating BMI (see opposite), the resulting number can be plotted on the standard BMI chart just as your child's height and weight are plotted on growth charts (see page 17).

Most children fall into the healthy weight category, which takes in a wide range of height and weight measurements. But BMI charts also can help doctors identify children who are overweight or at risk of becoming overweight. If spotted early, doctors and parents can work together to prevent a child from becoming overweight by helping the child make changes in exercise and eating habits.

The number of overweight children is increasing, so it is useful to calculate and plot BMI for your child on a regular basis. As with height and weight percentiles, this allows you and your GP to track the child's BMI over time.

Putting BMI in perspective

For most children BMI is a good indicator of body fat, but it is important to recognize that BMI is not a direct measurement of body fat. In fact, for some children and teenagers BMI values can be misleading. For example, muscle is significantly heavier than fat, so more muscular children may have high BMI scores even though their percentage of body fat may be in the healthy range. A muscular teenager could have a BMI in the overweight range, but probably does not have too much body fat.

On the other hand, a child can have an ideal BMI and still have too much body fat. And kids in the healthy weight range can be at risk of becoming overweight. Risk factors include a low level of physical activity, a diet high in fatty, sugary foods, and a family history of weight problems.

BMI also may be difficult to interpret during puberty when it's normal for girls and boys to gain weight and show dramatic increases in BMI. A parent may need a doctor's or nutritionist's help to judge whether a child's rapid weight gain is a normal part of maturation or if it warrants concern.

Some parents worry that their child is too thin or doesn't eat enough. But few children who are underweight on the growth charts turn out to have a health problem or other reason for concern. If you are worried about your child's low weight, talk with your GP. Never start a thin child on a high-calorie diet without consulting a doctor first. And, unless the low weight is related to an eating disorder such as anorexia nervosa or bulimia (see page 147), regular exercise should remain a healthy part of a child's routine.

What if my child is overweight?

When someone is overweight, genetic factors, lifestyle habits, or both are involved. Because both genes and habits can be passed down from one generation to the next, entire families may struggle with excess weight. You may be upset to learn that your child's BMI, weight, or the trend in weight gain is cause for concern. But identifying weight as a health concern can be the first step towards adopting new, healthier habits for your child and for the whole family.

For most overweight children, dieting is unnecessary and is not encouraged. You should never put your child on a slimming diet without a doctor's or dietitian's okay. Drastically reducing calories or cutting out foods containing essential nutrients may be dangerous to your child's health or interfere with overall growth and development. The goal with children should never be hitting a specific mark on the scale. Instead, the aim should be to help your child get into a weight range that allows healthy growth and development.

It's important that children learn the importance of healthy eating and exercise – without taking it too far. Be on the lookout for signs that they are taking the initiative to diet on their own. Many adolescents, especially young girls, feel uncomfortable with the normal weight gain that occurs with the onset of puberty. Help them understand these changes and be willing to answer questions. Educate them about the dangers of fad diets, fasting, and other dietary restrictions that may hurt their health and growth. (To learn about the symptoms of eating disorders, see page 163.)

Assessing your child's **BMI**

First calculate your child's BMI using one of the formulas below. Look for that number along the left side of the boys' or girls' chart, then find your child's age along the bottom. Draw your finger along the lines from these two points. Where the lines intersect in the chart is your child's weight category.

METRIC FORMULA

To calculate your child's BMI using metric measurements, use the mathematical formula:

BMI = weight in kg ÷ [height in m x height in m]

1 Multiply your child's height in metres by itself.

2 Use the result to divide his or her weight in kilograms.

IMPERIAL FORMULA

To calculate your child's BMI in Imperial measurements, use the mathematical formula:

BMI = [weight in lb ÷ height in in ÷ height in in] x 703

1 Divide your child's weight in pounds by his or her height in inches, divided by his or her height in inches.

2 Multiply the result by 703.

THE WEIGHT RANGES

Once you know your child's BMI you can plot it against his or her age on the BMI chart. The four weight ranges are:

- Underweight: below the shaded area
- Healthy weight: in the shaded area
- Overweight: just above the shaded area
- Obese: above the top line on the graph

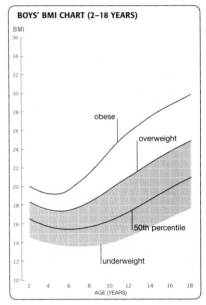

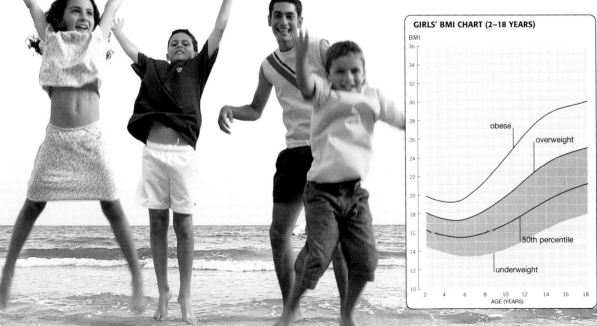

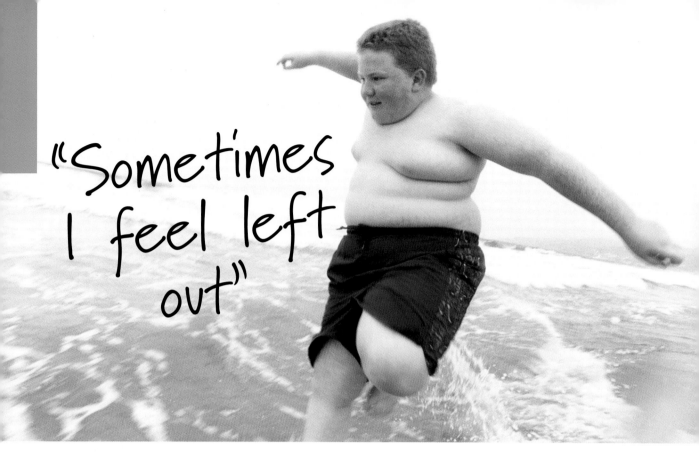

"Sometimes I feel left out"

Overweight children

Since 1980, the number of children who are overweight has increased threefold. Everyone wants to know why children are getting heavier and what needs to be done to stop this trend.

Problems ahead

In the UK today, the pattern of overweight and obesity in the young does not bode well. One in three children is overweight, and nine percent of two- to four-year-olds and 16 percent of six- to 15-year-olds are obese. That translates into a lot of kids and a lot of worried parents.

The best advice is: address the problem sooner rather than later. It's easier to help a four-year-old with a mild weight problem than a 12-year-old with a severe one. In fact, only 20 percent of overweight four-year-olds will become overweight adults, but 40 percent of seven-year-olds and up to 80 percent of teenagers who are overweight will become overweight adults.

The good news is that kids have a few advantages over adults when it comes to reaching a healthy weight. One main advantage is you: a concerned parent who wants to help. Children, especially pre-teens and younger, can be positively influenced by parents who steer them in the right direction when it comes to food and fitness. On top of that, kids burn a lot of calories just being kids. Their bodies are working hard to grow and most kids are naturally very active.

Ignoring a child's weight problem can increase the risk of serious medical conditions (for information about this, see page 22). The social and emotional consequences also can be severe, and can multiply and worsen if a heavy child grows into an overweight adult.

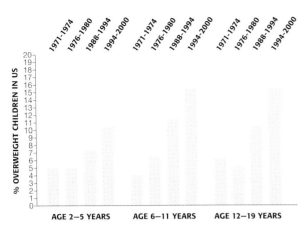

Rising number of overweight children
This chart shows the dramatic rise in the percentage of overweight children in the US. Health professionals in the UK are concerned that based on current statistics this trend is being repeated in Britain.

Emotional consequences

Overweight children often face social and emotional challenges. They may be ignored, teased, or viewed as unpopular by peers. As a result of social rejection, a child who is overweight may develop a negative self-image, which can undermine his or her feelings of self-worth and self-confidence. Social rejection based on weight becomes even more pronounced among adolescents. Exercise can help, but overweight children may be reluctant to exercise because they can't keep up or are embarrassed about how they look in shorts or fearful of changing clothes in front of other kids. For some overweight children, the social difficulties caused by their weight may trigger additional problems. Children who are unhappy with their weight and appearance are more likely to skip meals or try dangerous diets. Overweight children also may be more prone to depression and risky behaviours such as drug and alcohol use.

Medical consequences

Paediatricians and family GPs are starting to treat children who have weight-related health problems previously seen only in adults: high blood pressure and Type 2 diabetes are now being diagnosed in overweight children. These are risk factors for cardiovascular disease in adults, but the seeds of these problems are often planted in childhood. In response, expert groups, including the Royal College of Physicians, Royal College of Paediatrics and Child Health, and the Faculty of Public Health Medicine, are urging doctors to take a more proactive approach to reducing the growing number of children with weight problems. Children who carry excess weight and resulting health problems into adulthood will be at increased risk of heart attack and stroke.

What is Type 2 diabetes?

Diabetes is a disease caused by the body being unable to produce enough of the hormone insulin. Insulin is needed to move sugar, used as fuel, from the bloodstream into the body's cells.

There are two principal types of diabetes: Type 1 and Type 2. With Type 1, the body is unable to produce any insulin at all and regular injections of the hormone are needed to keep blood sugar levels as normal as possible. The disease appears most commonly in young school-age children and teenagers. The risk for getting it runs in families and it is not related to weight. (For more information about Type 1 diabetes, see page 176.)

However, most people who get Type 2 diabetes are overweight. A person with Type 2 diabetes can continue to make insulin, but is unable to respond to it normally, a condition known as insulin resistance. As a result, oral medication and/or insulin injections may be needed.

Previously called adult-onset diabetes, Type 2 diabetes was until very recently unheard of in children and teenagers. But although it is still relatively rare in the UK – current figures suggest that there are less than 100 children with Type 2 diabetes – numbers are doubling every year. Doctors are also starting to see signs of insulin resistance in children as young as five.

Diabetes and insulin resistance increase the risk of developing heart disease, stroke, and kidney failure later in life. In addition, new evidence suggests that having Type 2 diabetes may increase the risk of developing Alzheimer's disease.

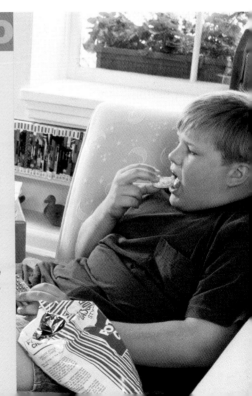

Common complaints

Although medical advances have improved children's health in many ways, there has been a rise in the number of overweight and obese children showing up in the doctor's surgery. Overweight children often do not feel as well as their peers and there are many possible explanations. Here are some common complaints:

"I'm the tallest in my class." Overweight boys and girls tend to grow faster and may enter puberty at an earlier age, making them taller and more sexually mature than their peers. This can be a burden because they may be expected to act as old as they look, not as old as they are. Overweight children who mature earlier, particularly girls, are more likely to carry their excess fat into adulthood.

"My knees hurt." Overweight children may have trouble with their bones and joints, and knee pain is a common complaint. It can deter a child from participating in PE class or other physical activities. Serious orthopaedic problems that require surgical treatment can occur in overweight children. Limping or complaints of pain in the knees, hips, or legs should be evaluated by a doctor.

"I'm so tired I fall asleep in class." Severe overweight contributes to restless or disordered sleep patterns including sleep apnoea, an interruption in breathing that disrupts sleep. When a child doesn't get enough sleep at night, it makes it difficult to pay attention during school hours. Sleep apnoea also can lower oxygen levels in the bloodstream, straining the heart and increasing blood pressure.

"I skip a lot of periods." Though overweight girls tend to enter puberty early, they may have irregular menstrual cycles due to hormonal imbalances. These girls may have fertility problems later, when they reach adulthood.

"I'm out of breath in PE class." Exercise can make an overweight child feel short of breath. For children who have asthma, weight gain can make symptoms worse. A doctor should be consulted if a child has any breathing problems.

Health problems associated with **being severely overweight**

As more children become overweight, weight-related health problems are being seen more frequently in the doctor's surgery. Some illnesses, such as Type 2 diabetes, are starting to affect kids during childhood. Other problems don't occur until adulthood, but the seeds are often planted because a person was overweight as a child. Likewise, the risk of these health problems can be lowered if a child maintains a healthy weight.

CHILDHOOD

- breathlessness
- asthma and other breathing problems
- sleep apnoea (pauses in breathing while asleep)
- high blood pressure
- Type 2 diabetes
- problems with knee and hip joints
- menstrual irregularities
- raised cholesterol
- liver disease
- gallstones and gall bladder disease
- depression

ADULT (LONG-TERM)

- high blood pressure
- raised cholesterol
- Type 2 diabetes
- cardiovascular problems (including heart attack and stroke)
- congestive heart failure
- respiratory problems, sleep apnoea
- higher risk of certain cancers (breast, prostate, colon)
- higher risk of sudden death
- higher risk of complications from anaesthesia and surgical procedures
- infertility and pregnancy complications
- arthritis
- liver disease
- gallstones and gall bladder disease
- gout
- depression

Getting help

Your child's doctor will evaluate the severity of any weight problem and may suggest a course of action. Options include a weight-management programme or referral to a dietitian, who will be able to guide you and your child towards appropriate nutrition goals.

A change in lifestyle

Your GP can recommend the steps you should take to help your overweight child. There are three possible approaches:
- slow the rate of weight gain;
- stop the weight gain;
- lose weight.

If your child is overweight, the goal will probably be to try to maintain a static weight so he or she becomes leaner as they grow in height. However, if your child is severely overweight or obese, weight loss will be part of the plan.

Any weight-loss regime should be supervised by a doctor or dietitian and should emphasize long-term lifestyle changes, not quick, short-term weight loss. Slimming diets – particularly those based on a very low calorie intake – and diet foods intended for adults are not appropriate for children. Also be wary of any children's weight-loss plan that makes unrealistic promises or guarantees results. (See page 147 for information about weight-loss camps.)

Expert advice

The doctor may refer you to a state-registered dietitian who can be a great resource for your family. A dietitian will evaluate your child's medical history and physical condition, including BMI measurements (see page 18). Using this information, the dietitian will suggest appropriate dietary changes as well as ways to help you and your child make them. She'll also recommend increased activity levels.

The diets of young children are easier to change because parents have greater control over food choices. Older children have to be trusted to follow the diet because they eat and spend more time away from home. This is why it is important for the older child himself or herself to be motivated to do something about their weight.

Work together

Parents need to remember that helping a child with a weight problem is a family affair, and must avoid laying down new food and fitness rules that apply only to the overweight child. Everyone will benefit from healthier habits, such as more nutritious meals, less TV time, and more exercise. Families who work together for healthier lifestyles have a better chance of success, so set achievable goals and celebrate the positive changes you're all making.

As you help your child, remember that it took time for him or her to gain the weight, and it will take time to make strides towards a healthier body. You can help your child most by setting a good example and, of course, by being a dependable source of encouragement, support, and love.

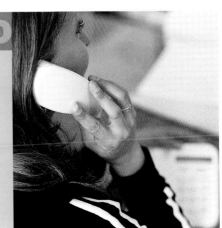

info

Consulting a dietitian

If you are worried about your child's weight, ask your GP to refer you to a state-registered dietitian (SRD). Growing children need a nutritionally balanced diet, with a good supply of essential nutrients like vitamins and minerals, to help them grow properly. Placing a child on a strict diet could easily lead to nutritional deficiencies, which could compromise his or her longer term health and growth. For this reason, it's very important to get advice from an appropriately qualified person before you place children on any sort of diet. Ask your GP or health visitor to make an appointment for you to see an SRD, who will be able to plan a diet suited to your child's individual needs.

Take a family approach

It may seem like an impossible dream to change your family's daily routine, but it's not. You can succeed by starting with small steps and everyone will benefit from adopting a healthier lifestyle.

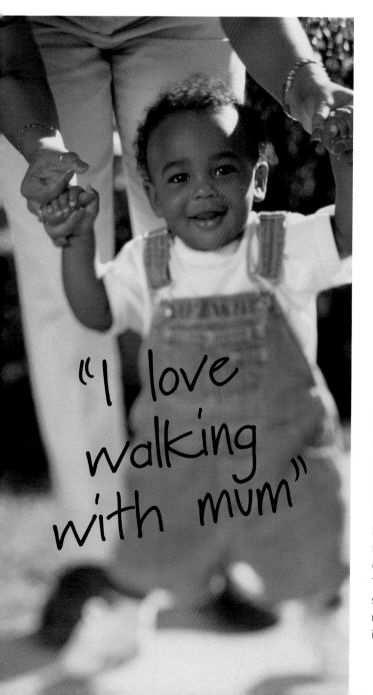

"I love walking with mum"

Team spirit

If you set out to change the way your family eats and exercises, expect a challenge. The process may lead you to re-examine and change some of your own habits. Stay the course, even when the going gets tough. The lessons you impart today about nutrition and fitness may become the healthy principles your child practises for a lifetime.

Involving the whole family is the best way to promote better eating and activity habits for your children. A whole-family approach simply means that everyone – parents and kids alike – works together as a team to achieve good health and well-being. As with any team, there's a leader or coach, and that's where you as a parent come in.

Lead by example Adult family members are important healthy eating and exercise role models. Talk about why you eat fruit as a snack, take an exercise class, or go for walks.

Start them young Don't wait until your child is overweight to institute good eating and activity habits. It's much easier to maintain a healthy weight than to lose excess later.

Be active together Make it usual for the family to be active, not sedentary. Being active as a family allows kids to expend energy in a positive way. Adults reap benefits too.

Cook together It may be impractical to do it every day, but invite children into the process of preparing food. Little kids can learn maths skills by measuring and they'll begin to understand the chemistry of cooking. They'll also gain an understanding of healthy ingredients. Older kids will enjoy having the authority to select and prepare foods they like. It may even inspire them to eat healthily on their own.

Eat together Eating a meal as a family sends the right messages about nutrition. Children will see their parents eating healthy food and may be inspired to try new foods. They will also come to see mealtime as an opportunity for socializing and sharing. Parents get a chance to offer nutritious food, note their child's likes and dislikes, and tune into their child's triumphs and troubles through conversation.

Family **goal chart**

Keeping a chart can remind family members to pay attention to eating and exercise habits. Choose family goals, such as exercising every day and eating fruits and vegetables, then keep track of who meets those goals. Keeping a chart can remind family members to pay attention to eating and exercise habits.

DAY	EXERCISED TODAY					ATE FRUIT AND VEG TODAY				
	MUM	DAD	JIM	EMILY	MIKE	MUM	DAD	JIM	EMILY	MIKE
Monday	✓	–	✓	✓	–	✓	–	✓	✓	✓
Tuesday	–	–	✓	–	✓	✓	✓	✓	–	✓
Wednesday	✓	✓	–	✓	✓	✓	✓	–	✓	✓
Thursday	–	✓	✓	✓	✓	–	✓	–	✓	✓
Friday	✓	–	–	✓	–	✓	✓	✓	–	✓
Saturday	–	–	✓	–	–	✓	–	✓	–	–
Sunday	✓	✓	✓	–	✓	✓	–	✓	✓	✓

tips

Family-friendly activities

If your family is prone to turning on the TV to relax, get out of your remote-control rut by trying these activities around the house.

Morning madness Does the sound of cartoons overwhelm your family breakfast? Instead of turning on the TV before you serve the toast, do some simple stretches or exercises with your child to get the blood flowing. Jumping up and down and running in place will be sure to wake you up.

Task force All family members can get involved in household tasks appropriate for their age. This not only results in more activity, your house will look better too.

Rainy day resolutions When it's raining hard outside, it's all too easy to let the TV take over. Instead, plan ahead by creating a rainy-day box filled with toys and games that your children can use only on those particularly wet days.

Blow off some steam Before settling in for evening activities or before dinner, take time to unwind together from a long day at school, home, or work. Play a quick game of tag or catch in the garden for an early evening boost.

Dance for your dinner While preparing dinner, put on some favourite tunes. Your child can move about while you cook.

Jump on a hobby horse Teach your child the basics of your favourite hobby, be it woodturning or making a scrapbook, and work on simple projects with him or her. They'll love the time spent with you.

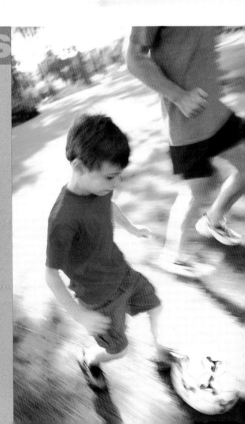

Raising a healthy eater

Healthy, positive attitudes about nutrition can be a lifelong gift you give to your children – and yourself. Remember that your kids will be influenced by the choices you make when you shop for food, cook family meals, and eat out in restaurants.

A nutritious, varied diet

Good nutrition in childhood is essential for optimal growth and development. It also:

- helps children maintain a healthy weight;
- provides fuel for learning and physical activity;
- encourages healthy eating habits that will serve them well throughout their lives.

Some parents wonder if they need to give their child vitamins. For most children, vitamin supplements are not necessary if they eat a variety of foods. The quantities of vitamin-rich foods don't have to be huge: with just half an orange, a five-year-old can meet the daily requirement for vitamin C. For a ten-year-old, a few baby carrots can meet the daily need for vitamin A. (See page 39 for more about vitamins and what they do.)

myth: **Eating healthy meals means throwing away cherished family recipes.**

fact: You can lighten up your family's fare without fuss, using these food substitution ideas. Try a small amount of the substitute first, then gradually increase the amount to ensure that you maintain the consistency and texture of the original ingredient. Your family members will never know the difference!

- Replace cream in puddings, sauces, and casseroles with evaporated skimmed milk.
- Cut the amount of oil in half when sautéeing.
- Substitute apple, prune, or apricot purée for oil and butter in baked goods.
- Try chicken stock to moisten mashed potatoes rather than butter.
- Make salad dressings and marinades with fruit juice rather than oil.
- Use cocoa powder in place of chocolate in cake and biscuit recipes.

Here are three simple guidelines for serving wholesome and nutritious food to your children:

- Offer plenty of fruits, vegetables, and whole-grain breads and cereals.
- Serve a variety of lower-fat protein foods, such as poultry, lean meat, tofu, fish, and eggs (see page 35 for more about protein).
- Encourage your children to drink water or milk instead of empty-calorie fizzy drinks.

In addition to offering healthy foods, parents can raise healthy eaters by teaching them to listen to their body's own hunger cues. This begins in infancy, believe it or not – even a baby will send signals that he or she is full by turning away from the bottle or breast.

As children get older, parents can continue to educate them about what their bodies are saying about feeling hungry or full. Responding to the body's hunger cues is a vital skill in maintaining a healthy weight.

Healthy shopping tips

You may think that it costs more to eat healthy foods, but in fact healthy, basic foods give you more value for money than a basketful of unhealthy snacks and ready meals.

- When you sit down to write your shopping list, focus your week's menus on wholesome, nutritious ingredients, such as fresh and frozen fruits and vegetables, lean meats and poultry, fresh fish, whole grains, and low-fat dairy products. Be sure to shop for healthy lunchbox and snack foods too.
- To save money, choose produce that's in season.
- Visit farmers' markets in your area for the best that local growers have to offer.
- When you're at the supermarket, try to stick to your shopping list. Don't be tempted by special offers on less healthy prepared foods and snacks that you know your family shouldn't really be eating.

For more information about healthy food shopping and reading food labels, see pages 46–48.

Don't take the hard line

If you get completely swept up in your lifestyle overhaul, you might be tempted to declare a ban on all foods that contain sugar or chocolate, or that are high in fat. Don't do it. Completely eliminating sweets and favourite snacks can backfire if your child feels deprived. The result could be that your child overeats the off-limits food whenever given the opportunity outside the home.

Instead of taking the hard line or completely giving in, strive for moderation. Try not to talk about "bad foods". Don't be afraid to allow your child to choose a treat when shopping. You could even bake a special dessert together. But set limits. For example, fill a small bowl with tortilla chips to satisfy a snack craving, rather than leaving the whole bag out. This is enough to meet your child's desire for a sweet or crunchy snack food while still allowing room for healthier foods.

Dining out

With busy schedules, many families turn to restaurants for quick and easy meals. But it's no secret that in some restaurants the portions can be quite large. When there's no time to cook at home, try to use restaurant food wisely.

When eating at restaurants, don't limit your children to a kids' menu, which usually offers things like chips and chicken nuggets. Instead, look for healthier choices on the regular menu and ask if you can get a child's portion of an adult meal. If not, given the size of most main courses, you might be able to split the meal between two children, or you could share the meal with your child. If that meal includes a salad or vegetable, all the better. You also might consider getting a take-away so you can order fewer main dishes, and serve the meal family-style at home.

If you find yourself ordering a take-away, at the window of a drive-through restaurant or queueing at a fast-food counter, you're not alone. In the UK there's been a dramatic increase in the consumption of fast food: in 2001 around two billion meals were eaten at "quick service" food outlets.

But even fast food can be managed through moderation. For example, let your child have a burger and chips once in a while, just not every day or every week. If fast food is the only option, be a role model with your own order. Fast food restaurants are expanding their menu of lower-fat alternatives, which means you can opt for grilled chicken, salad, yogurt, or soup. Your child might follow your lead next time.

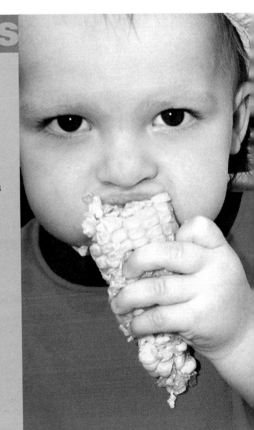

tips

Dos and don'ts for healthy eating

- Do allow your children to eat according to their hunger signals. Listen to them when they say they're hungry, and allow them to stop eating when they indicate their hunger is satisfied.
- Do help your child cultivate an adventurous approach to different food tastes and textures.
- Do ensure your child eats plenty of whole grains, fruits, and vegetables to promote digestive health.
- Do provide structured eating and snacking times each day, based on regular meals and snacks.
- Do limit eating at fast-food restaurants.
- Do eat together as a family and offer nutritious choices.
- Do take your time at family meals. Eating slowly allows your child time to digest the food and register a sense of fullness.

- Don't offer dessert or any other sweet treat as a reward for finishing a meal (or to reward anything else).
- Don't use food as an incentive or for stress and boredom relief. Food is easily associated with soothing hurt feelings, nurturing, and comfort, but it's important to help children learn other ways of comforting themselves so that they do not become dependent on food for this.
- Don't force your child to eat everything that's served. Did your parents admonish you to "clean your plate" because "children are starving in other countries"? Past attitudes towards eating may have focused on reducing waste, but that may lead to unhealthy habits because it puts children out of touch with their hunger signals.
- Don't eat in front of the television.

Raising an active child

From an early age, children enjoy moving their bodies. The trick for parents is to foster and encourage that natural love of activity so children can reap the physical, emotional, and social benefits of regular exercise as they grow older.

Instil positive fitness habits

Active children develop self-confidence, feel more in control of their bodies, and are less likely to be overweight. Through activity, they learn balance and coordination, burn calories, and build muscle. And, just like adults, exercise allows children to relieve stress. So when they are young, start a routine of family-centred fitness. Initially, this may seem like an unproductive way to spend a few hours, but it's an excellent strategy for instilling positive fitness habits. Those habits may be very beneficial later on, when it's tempting for children to drop exercise in favour of sedentary activities. The time you spend learning a new sport together or walking in the park is also an opportunity to connect with your child.

Many ways to be active

You'll want to select activities that are appropriate for your child's age. (Turn to the age-specific chapters for help with this.) It's not reasonable, for instance, to expect a three-year-old to complete a 24-km (15-mile) bike ride. Also, if you have children who span a range of ages, you'll need to find an activity that will work for everyone.

Let your children explore different ways of being active by taking lessons to learn new sports and joining teams to get regular practice sessions. Seek out non-competitive sports for young children and for those who dislike the pressure of competition. Be sensitive to your child's likes and dislikes. Some may choose solitary pursuits such as running or swimming over team sports.

If a child doesn't want to do something or doesn't seem ready, it's best not to push too hard. Children develop skills at different ages (see more about this on page 54) and should be allowed to progress at their own pace. Also remember that a child's interests will grow and change over the years. A three-year-old may be happy to play catch in the garden, but a young school-age child might be more interested in a game of hopscotch. And in the teenage years, hopscotch will seem too childish, so your adolescent may want to take a yoga class or join a basketball team.

Rationing the TV and computer

Regular physical activity is only one piece of the puzzle. Another key strategy is to limit the amount of time family members spend in sedentary activities. Some experts say

A natural mood-lifter
Everyone can reap the benefits of getting exercise. And just like family meals, family exercise is a good chance for parents and children to connect with each other.

myth: **Your child needs at least an hour of vigorous exercise to reap any benefit.**

fact: The consensus is that your child doesn't need to run for an hour on the treadmill each night to be physically fit. But starting in the pre-school years, children need 30–60 minutes of physical activity every day, such as playing games in the garden or going for a walk. They also need an hour or more of free play every day. In addition to being active every day, teenagers need to get some vigorous physical activity. A good recommendation is at least three 20-minute sessions a week.

parents should not allow children under age two to watch any TV or videos, and that all children over age two (and that includes teenagers) should spend no more than one to two hours a day watching TV and playing computer games.

Aside from being sedentary, watching TV can have other negative effects. Commercial TV allows advertisers to target kids' shows with advertisements for high-sugar and high-fat foods – it's no coincidence that children often snack in front of the TV. Try to offer them healthy snacks (or, better still, avoid associating TV-watching with eating altogether!).

Fitting in fitness

Though it may seem trivial, seize everyday opportunities to get a little more activity yourself. You may be surprised how easy it is to fit some simple exercise into your daily routine.

- Take the stairs, not the lift or escalator.
- If it's feasible, walk, instead of driving, to a friend's house or a nearby shop.
- On shopping trips, try to walk briskly, to get the blood pumping, rather than stroll from store to store.
- Instead of circling the car park looking for a close space, choose a spot farther away from the supermarket or your office and get in a brief but brisk walk.
- If your child's school is close enough, walk or bike your child there and back.
- When doing household tasks, get the whole family involved, and get everybody moving energetically.

Finally, don't neglect your own health. When you act as a positive role model for your child, it shows him or her that fitness isn't just for children – it's about being healthy for life. Make time for exercise several times each week and let your child see that exercise is a priority for you too.

tips

Ideas for outings

Are you stumped as to what to do for your next family outing? Here are some tips for keeping your family interested in fitness:

Make it kid's choice Maybe your child is clamouring for a game of cricket in the local park, even though you've planned a walk. Letting your child choose the family activity encourages physical fitness and helps him or her develop self-confidence.

Now we're getting somewhere Let your child research how many kilometres it is to a city he or she would like to visit. Then, every time you walk a kilometre as a family, record it. When you've "walked" as far as the destination, reward your child with a special toy or activity – or go there.

Won't you be my neighbour? You don't have to drive somewhere to get active – organize a neighbourhood football, cricket, or rounders game with the other families in your area.

Sign up the family for a fun run Or try training for a bike race. The thrill of competing together as a family is one of the best ways to cement everybody's commitment to fitness.

Give back Volunteering can be a great way to get out and get active. Look for local opportunities for your family to spend time outdoors – check with your local community centre or library or the local authority recreation department for ideas.

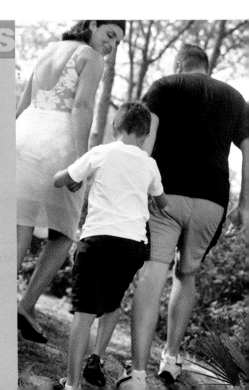

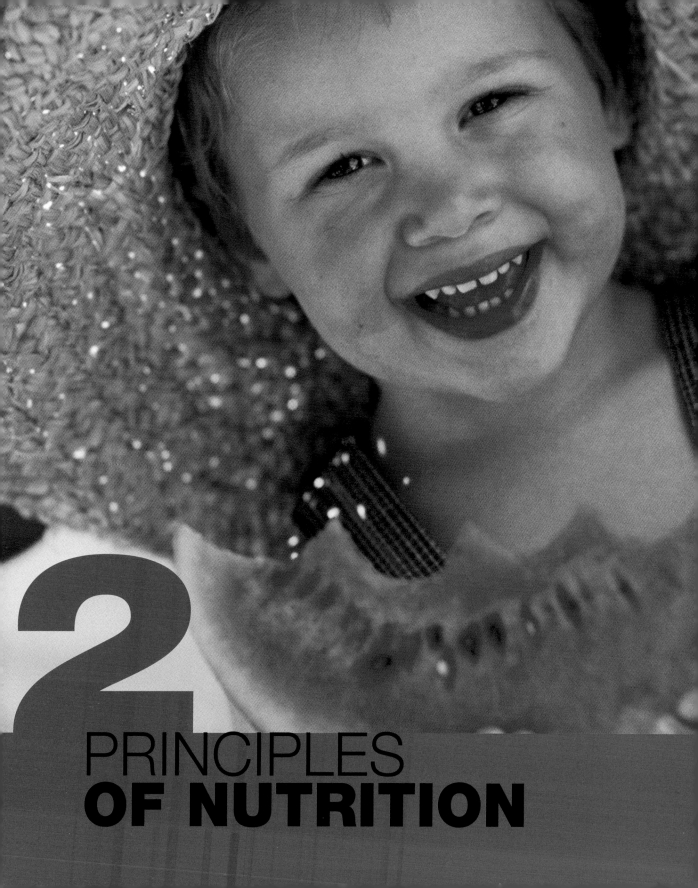

2
PRINCIPLES
OF NUTRITION

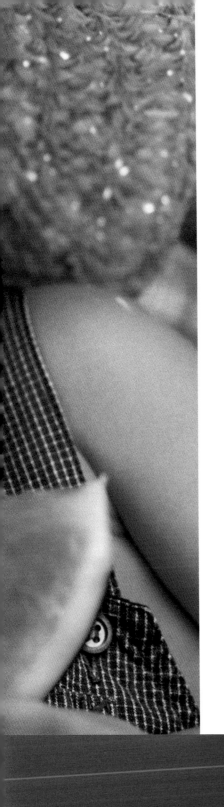

If you want to **help your child eat well**, all you need to do is serve healthy foods that have the **nutrients kids need to grow** and develop. Don't argue with your child over food. **Be flexible** – but in a smart way.

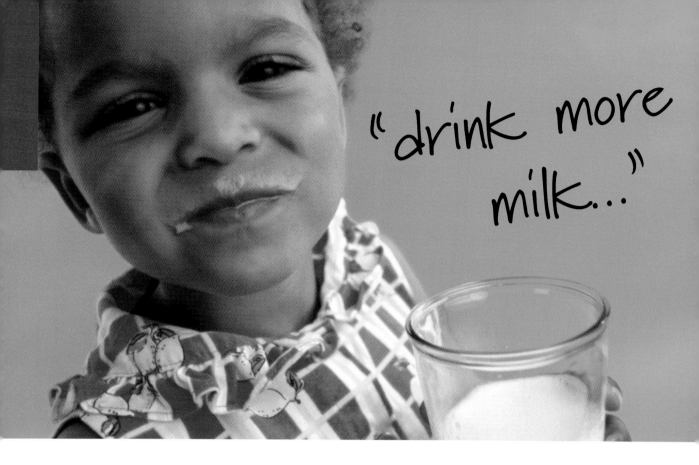

"drink more milk..."

The vital components of food

Each family's diet will vary according to tradition and personal preferences, but the building blocks of a healthy and nutritious way of eating are the same for everyone.

What we need and how to get it

Our bodies – and especially the growing bodies of children – rely on carbohydrates, fibre, protein, fat, vitamins, and minerals, as well as water. We obtain these from the food we eat. In the right amounts, these nutrients provide the basis of good health and vitality.

It's easy to be confused about good nutrition for children and to get lost in all the recommended guidelines. It can be difficult to understand why your infant needs almost half of his or her calories from fat while your six-year-old would be better off with only a third from fat and more calories from carbohydrate foods (see chart, opposite). Meanwhile, you have to ensure that your 11-year-old daughter has the

calcium she needs – which is more than her younger brother requires (see page 38). And if your child is a bit fussy, you may be wondering how you can keep everything in balance with only pizza and tuna sandwiches. Happily, you don't need a degree in nutrition science to feed your child a healthy diet. You just need to understand some basic principles and to adopt a few healthy habits – habits that will be good for the whole family.

The recommended daily amounts (RDAs) for individual nutrients, serving sizes, and grams per day are useful guidelines, but can be difficult to track. It's reassuring to know that you can achieve good results by striving for a diet full of variety, colour, and, of course, fun!

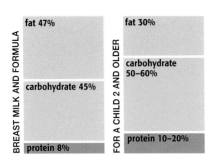

BREAST MILK AND FORMULA
fat 47%
carbohydrate 45%
protein 8%

FOR A CHILD 2 AND OLDER
fat 30%
carbohydrate 50–60%
protein 10–20%

Changing requirements
A diet of breast milk or formula gives a baby plenty of fat to fuel growth. Between 12 and 24 months, the diet should change gradually to include more protein and carbohydrates, and less fat.

Why variety?

Children who eat a wide assortment of foods increase their chances of meeting their nutritional requirements. Serve foods from all the food groups: carbohydrate foods, dairy products, meat and other protein foods, fruits, and vegetables (for more about the food groups, see page 40).

Why colour?

A colourful plate typically contains a good range of nutrients and also looks very appetizing. Here's a tempting example: red salsa and green guacamole alongside a wrap filled with chicken, red onion, green pepper, and yellow courgettes. This provides protein, carbohydrate, fat, vitamins A and C, folate, potassium, and calcium.

Why fun?

Whether your child is seven months, seven years, or 17, food should be a shared source of enjoyment. It's important that children see food as a pleasure, so don't force them to clean their plates or eat foods they dislike. This doesn't mean they should get to pick alternative meals or alternative mealtimes. It just means letting them choose how much to eat from the variety of healthy foods you make available. Let toddlers feed themselves, even if it's a bit messy. Tempt pre-school children with a vegetable smile on top of a pizza. Encourage older children to help prepare dishes. And congratulate all children when they try new foods.

It averages out

Nutrition is all about averages. Not getting enough of one nutrient on one day isn't a problem if your child gets enough on most days – it all balances out. In fact, meeting daily nutritional requirements is easier than you might think. With just 75g (2½oz) of cooked broccoli, a four- to eight-year-old child would get 25 percent of daily fibre needs, 12 percent of the RDA for iron, 6 percent of the RDA for calcium, and more than 100 percent of the RDA for vitamin C.

Some of you may be thinking: "My child won't touch broccoli!" It is true that the child who will eat only a few foods does create a challenge. But even fussy eaters can meet their nutritional requirements without parents pleading or arguing about their eating habits. The good news is that fussiness can be just a phase.

The best ways to make children eat healthily – whether they are fussy or easy-going about eating – are to have plenty of healthy food choices available and to be a good role model by eating them yourself. By doing this, you'll increase the chances that when hunger strikes, your child will reach for something nutritious, even if you're not there.

Calories in, energy out

A calorie is a unit of energy. It is so small that when we use the term calorie we actually mean a kilocalorie (kcal), which is equivalent to 1000 true calories.

The number of calories in a serving of food indicates how much energy that food gives the body. The components of food contain differing amounts of calories:
● 1g fat provides 9 calories.
● 1g carbohydrate provides 4 calories.
● 1g protein provides 4 calories.
Naturally, children's calorie requirements vary with weight, age, and activity level.

These figures for calorie requirements per day assume normal activity:
● Toddlers: 1000–1200 calories
● Pre-school kids: 1200–1600 calories
● School-age kids: 1600–2200 calories
● Adolescent girls: 1845–2110 calories
● Adolescent boys: 2200–2750 calories
We are conditioned to try to avoid calories, to prevent weight gain, but they are necessary for the body to function and grow. Calories become a problem only when people take in more calories than they are able to burn off.

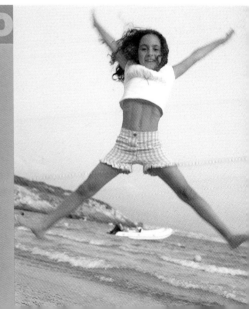

Carbohydrates

Both adults and children need carbohydrates, which are the body's most important and readily available source of energy. (See the age-specific chapters for carbohydrate needs.)

Most foods contain carbohydrates. The two major forms of carbohydrates are simple sugars (simple carbohydrates) and starches (complex carbohydrates), which are broken down into simple sugars when digested. So foods containing carbohydrates – be they complex (found in breads, cereals, rice, pasta, and starchy vegetables) or simple (sugars, such as fructose, glucose, and lactose) – are not bad for you. But some carbohydrate foods are healthier choices than others.

- Complex carbohydrate foods, such as unrefined grains, brown rice, and whole-grain breads and cereals, are packed with nutrients. They're broken down more slowly in the body and are high in fibre, so are filling enough to discourage overeating. Whole fruits contain simple sugars but have the added benefit of vitamins and fibre.
- Simple carbohydrates, especially refined sugars and more refined grains, such as white rice and white flour, have been stripped of vitamins and minerals. These low-fibre carbohydrates are easy to overeat because they aren't very filling. Simple carbohydrates like sugar provide what nutritionists call "empty calories" – calories that offer nothing else in the way of nutrients.

When carbohydrates are eaten, the simple sugars released during digestion are absorbed into the blood stream. As the sugar level rises, the pancreas releases the hormone insulin, which is necessary for moving sugar from the blood into the cells where the sugar can be used as a source of energy.

For decades, scientists have known that different foods, even if they contain the same amount of carbohydrate, don't cause the same rise in blood sugar (and insulin level). This is related to the specific types of carbohydrate in the food, the fibre content, and other factors that affect the way carbohydrates are digested and absorbed. To measure these differences, foods can be analyzed using the glycaemic index (see below).

Scientists have been investigating the possible relationship between carbohydrates and the risk of developing diseases such as diabetes and heart disease. Some studies suggest there is an increased risk among people who eat a diet high in foods that cause a greater rise in blood sugar. It's thought that the higher insulin levels in the blood triggered by these foods may play a key role in the increased risk of disease.

Fibre

Everyone needs fibre, which moves food through the digestive system, fighting constipation. It adds no calories, yet makes us feel full. It may lower LDL-cholesterol ("bad" cholesterol) levels and help prevent diabetes and heart disease.

Fibre is found in plants – fruits, vegetables, and grains. Food made from plant products, such as breads and cereals, as well as fruits and vegetables, provides fibre. Whole-grain breads and cereals contain more than white bread and white rice. Some of the best fruit and vegetable sources are apples, berries, prunes, broccoli, carrots, peas, and beans.

For pre-school children, an increase in fibre intake should be done gradually. Too much fibre can make a young child's diet so bulky that he or she becomes full before eating sufficient food to satisfy essential nutrient needs.

Q: What is the glycaemic index?

A: Over the past 20 years, researchers have developed a standardized method of evaluating how the body handles different carbohydrates in foods. Called the glycaemic index (GI), this measure compares the rise in blood sugar that occurs after eating a particular food with the rise in blood sugar that occurs after eating the same amount of carbohydrate in a standard food (usually white bread). The higher the spike in blood sugar, compared to the bread, the higher the food's glycaemic index will be.

Because foods with a low GI are thought to be healthier, magazines and books are now promoting the virtues of a low-glycaemic-index diet. But the findings of scientific studies, which have been done mostly on adults, are still being debated and everyone agrees that more research is needed. What does all this mean when deciding what to feed your child? You're already on safe ground if you're limiting simple sugars and foods made from refined flours and grains. These are also the ones with the highest GI. Opt instead for more high-fibre, nutrient-rich carbohydrate foods, such as fruits, vegetables, and whole grains. These foods have health benefits for children – and most have a low GI.

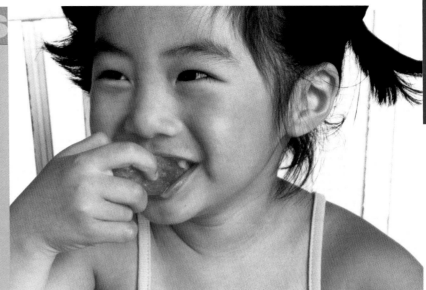

tips

Easy ways to get more fibre

- Leave skins on fruits and vegetables.
- Sprinkle wheat germ on breakfast cereal or yogurt.
- Add some bran to the mixture for a meat loaf or burgers.
- Offer raisins as snacks or add them to salads.
- Serve brown rice and wholemeal spaghetti and other pasta.
- Substitute wholemeal flour for some of the white flour when baking bread, cakes, and so on.

A source of fibre is one that provides 3g or more per serving (a good source provides at least 6g). Bran cereals provide 3.5g fibre per bowl, a medium pear with skin provides 3.3g fibre, and 100g (3½oz) baked beans provides 3.7g fibre.

Protein

While carbohydrates provide fuel, proteins help build and repair essential parts of the body. Protein is found in meat, poultry, fish, eggs, dairy products, nuts, seeds, pulses, and grains. The body breaks protein down into components called amino acids, which are used to build and maintain muscles, bones, body organs, the blood, and the immune system.

Protein is key to healthy growth, so it's important for children to eat enough on a regular basis. Fortunately, in Britain few people get too little protein. You can figure out how much protein your child needs every day based on how much he or she weighs: the formula is approximately 1.0 gram of protein for every kilogram body weight (0.5 gram per pound). So a 25-kg (50-lb) child should have about 25g protein every day. These foods together would satisfy that daily requirement:

- 1 tablespoon peanut butter (4g protein);
- 240ml (8floz) semi-skimmed milk (8g protein);
- 30g (1oz) or two domino-sized pieces of Cheddar cheese (7g protein);
- 30g (1oz) or a matchbox-sized piece of baked chicken breast (7g protein).

Protein from animal sources, including milk products, is called "complete" because it contains all nine of the essential amino acids. Vegetable protein is considered "incomplete" because it lacks one or more of the essential amino acids. This can be a concern for someone following a vegetarian diet, but you can create a complete protein by combining different proteins that together provide all nine essential amino acids. This isn't hard to do: peanut butter with whole-grain bread, and kidney beans with rice are just two examples. And you don't have to make the right combinations at every meal as long as you eat a variety of foods throughout the day.

Fat

An adequate fat intake is essential to growth and development. Fats fuel the body and aid in the absorption of some vitamins. They are the building blocks of hormones and are necessary for insulating all nervous system tissue in the body.

There is disagreement among nutrition experts about the amount of fat that should be in a healthy diet, for both children and adults. It is true that fat has more than twice as many calories as protein or carbohydrates (see page 33), but some experts think the low-fat revolution has gone too far, overlooking the complex nature of fats and how they work in the body. For one thing, eating fat in a meal helps us feel more satisfied, so we may be less likely to overeat. And replacing fat calories with simple sugars in a low-fat diet can have negative effects on health as well.

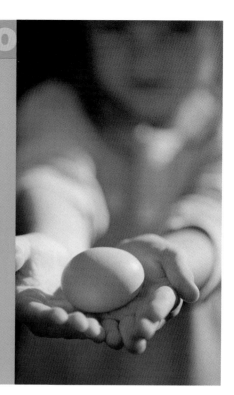

info

What's the story on cholesterol?

Cholesterol has a negative image, but it's a necessary component of cells. There are two sources:

- foods such as meat, whole milk, and egg yolks (dietary cholesterol);
- cholesterol manufactured by the body in the liver.

Blood cholesterol exists in two major forms: HDL (the "good" type) and LDL (the "bad" one). Too much LDL in the bloodstream increases the risk of heart disease as it can collect in the arteries and block them. HDL gets carried out of the bloodstream to be recycled and used elsewhere in the body.

Genes play an important role in how the body handles cholesterol and dietary fat. When children inherit a tendency to produce too much LDL and/or too little HDL, they have a higher risk of developing heart disease as they grow older. Eating the right balance of dietary fats is thought to be important for helping reduce this risk.

It used to be thought that avoiding foods high in dietary cholesterol was the answer, but the quantity of cholesterol you eat is not a major factor in determining how much ends up in your bloodstream: now it is known that saturated fat and trans fats tend to raise the levels of LDL in the blood. This is true for children as well as for adults, so it's wise to begin watching your child's intake of saturated and trans fats from age two onwards. Serve whole milk and red meat only occasionally. Instead opt for chicken, nuts, and other foods that contain the healthier unsaturated fats.

There are different types of fat

"Adequate" fat doesn't mean unlimited – too much can be a problem, as can the kind of fat you eat. The major types are:

Unsaturated fats: found in plant foods and fish. These fats are seen as neutral or even beneficial to heart health. Some of the healthiest include monounsaturated fats (found in olive, and groundnut oils and in avocados), polyunsaturated fats (found in most vegetable oils), and omega-3 fatty acids (from oily fish such as fresh tuna, pilchards, and sardines).

Saturated fat: found in animal products including meat, lard, butter, cheese, and milk (except skimmed milk) as well as in palm and coconut oils. A high intake of saturated fat raises blood cholesterol levels in some people and is a risk factor for heart disease (see above).

Trans fats: found in some margarines and commercial snack foods, pastry, cakes, and biscuits. Trans fats are created when vegetable oils are hydrogenated (so they remain solid at room temperature). A high intake can pose the same risks to health as saturated fats. Trans fats don't have to be noted on food labels, but if a product lists "hydrogenated" or "partially hydrogenated" fats in the ingredients, you can assume it contains trans fats. (For more information, see page 48.)

Water

Children – and adults – need water, but as water is found in foods such as fruits and drinks other than water like milk, there's no guideline for how much water kids should drink. A healthy child's body does a good job of regulating fluid and children tend to drink when they're thirsty. But what about those who are too young to tell you they're thirsty?

Under normal circumstances, infants don't need water. Giving them water may diminish their hunger and keep them from getting the nutrients provided by breast milk or formula. But older children can and should drink water, particularly as an alternative to sugary and fizzy drinks.

When children are out in hot weather, offer extra fluids. Be sure they get a drink before, during, and after exercising too. (See page 67 for information about dehydration.) The availability of bottled water makes this easy, but a sports bottle you can refill is a cheaper option – wash it with hot soapy water or put it in the dishwasher between uses.

The best drink

If offered water – or diluted fruit juice – from a young age, children are more likely to keep drinking water as they get older, rather than sugary, empty-calorie drinks.

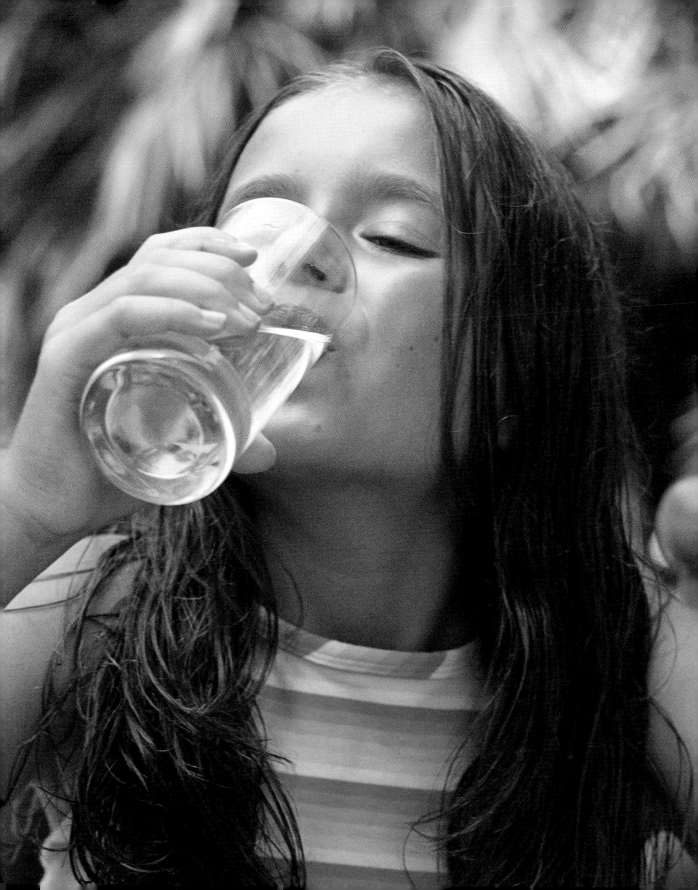

Vitamins and minerals

These substances serve critical functions in a child's growing body. Among their many roles, vitamins help with growth and development, and aid the functioning of organs and cells in normal metabolic processes.

Vitamins are found naturally in foods from animal or plant sources. In addition, children may get vitamins through vitamin-enriched foods such as cereals or juices. Because different vitamins act on different parts and processes of the body, a healthy diet includes all the essential vitamins, from A to K. Each one offers its own benefits.

Minerals such as calcium, potassium, and zinc fulfil a wide range of vital needs. Unlike vitamins, minerals are inorganic – they are not produced in plants or animals. Instead, plants and animals pick up minerals through what they absorb or eat, and we get them in turn from the plants or meat that we eat.

Deficiencies

Although vitamin and mineral deficiencies are uncommon in the UK, because most people eat a varied diet and many foods are enriched with nutrients, two deficiencies that are prevalent are iron and calcium. Iron deficiency can lead to

anaemia (when the oxygen-carrying pigment, haemoglobin, in red blood cells is low), as well as behavioural and learning problems in young children. Calcium deficiency increases the risk of osteoporosis, or brittle bone disease, in adulthood. Here are the daily recommendations for iron intake:

- birth to three months: 1.7mg
- four to six months: 4.3mg
- seven to 12 months: 7.8mg
- one to three years: 6.9mg
- four to six years: 6.1mg
- seven to ten years: 8.7mg
- 11–18 years: 11.3mg (boys), 14.8mg (girls)

These are the daily calcium requirements:

- birth to 12 months: 525mg
- one to three years: 350mg
- four to six years: 450mg
- seven to ten years: 550mg
- 11–18 years: 1000mg (boys), 800mg (girls)

Certain diets can put a child at increased risk of deficiency. For example, a vegetarian who doesn't eat meat, poultry, or fish may not get enough iron. A very low-fat diet may prevent absorption of fat-soluble vitamins such as vitamin A.

One vitamin deficiency has less to do with the foods you eat than with how much time you spend outdoors: when the skin is exposed to sun, the body makes vitamin D. You can also get vitamin D in foods such as fish and fortified milk.

Too much sodium

Sodium, a component of table salt, is essential for life. It plays an important role in maintaining water balance in the body and is needed to send nerve signals and contract muscles, including the heart. But we are getting too much salt in our diets, which can contribute to the development of high blood pressure. Experts now recommend that both adults and children need to cut down salt intake, and official daily limits for salt have now been issued for children: for toddlers 2g, for four- to six-year-olds 3g, for seven- to ten-year-olds 5g, and for children over 11 (and adults) 6g.

When shopping, read food labels to check salt or sodium content (1g of sodium is equal to 2.5g of salt) and shy away from highly processed foods such as salty snacks and soups. Also be careful about the amount of salt you add when cooking and limit the use of salt at the table. Aim to serve your family a diet rich in whole grains, fresh fruits, and vegetables, all foods that are naturally low in sodium.

Q: Does my child need vitamin supplements?

A: In general, children who eat a balanced diet and who do not have special health concerns do not need vitamin or mineral supplements. There are a couple of instances, however, when a doctor may suggest supplements:

- Babies who are breastfed are often prescribed drops with iron and fluoride supplements, and sometimes vitamins A, C, and D as well.
- Adolescents who don't drink milk may need calcium supplements to promote the growth of strong bones.
- Though fussy eaters usually get enough nutrients, giving a child a daily multivitamin may reassure some parents.

If you think your child needs a vitamin or mineral supplement, talk with your GP or health visitor. The safest supplements are multivitamins formulated for kids. Giving doses of individual vitamins and minerals can be very dangerous and lead to fatal overdoses.

Vitamins and minerals, and what they do

VITAMIN OR MINERAL	ESSENTIAL FOR	FOUND IN
Vitamin A (retinol)	healthy eyes, skin, teeth, bones	eggs, milk and dairy, liver; carotenoids, which the body converts into vitamin A, are found in fruits and vegetables, including carrots, sweet potatoes, orange-fleshed melon, dark green vegetables such as spinach
Vitamins B$_1$ (thiamin), B$_2$ (riboflavin), B$_3$ (niacin), and B$_6$	turning food into energy; maintaining nerves, muscles, skin, the digestive system, other structures; formation of red blood cells	whole grains, fish, pulses, nuts, eggs, enriched cereals, meats
Folate, the naturally occurring form of folic acid	formation of red blood cells and DNA, which contains the building plans for all cells	whole grains, green leafy vegetables, pulses, citrus fruits, poultry, pork, enriched breads and cereals
Vitamin B$_{12}$	central nervous system; formation of red blood cells	poultry, eggs, meat, seafood, dairy products
Vitamin C (ascorbic acid)	absorption of iron; sustaining healthy tissues; helping heal wounds	citrus fruits, orange-fleshed melon, strawberries, tomatoes, broccoli, cabbage
Vitamin D	calcium absorption; normal bone growth and maintenance	fortified dairy products, fish, egg yolks
Vitamin E	formation of red blood cells; maintenance of body tissues	whole grains, wheat germ, leafy green vegetables, sardines, egg yolks, nuts
Vitamin K	blood clotting	leafy green vegetables, liver, pork, dairy products
Calcium	teeth and bones; transmission of nerve signals; muscle contraction; control of hormone secretion	dairy products, canned salmon and sardines (with bones), green leafy vegetables such as broccoli, spring greens, pak choi, kale
Iron	formation of haemoglobin, which carries oxygen to tissues throughout the body	red meat, dark poultry, tuna, salmon, eggs, pulses, dried fruits, leafy green vegetables, whole grains
Potassium	muscle and nervous system function; maintaining the balance of water in the blood and body tissues	broccoli, potatoes (with skins), leafy green vegetables, citrus fruits, bananas, dried fruits, pulses
Zinc	immune system function; cell growth; wound healing	beef, pork, lamb, peanuts, pulses

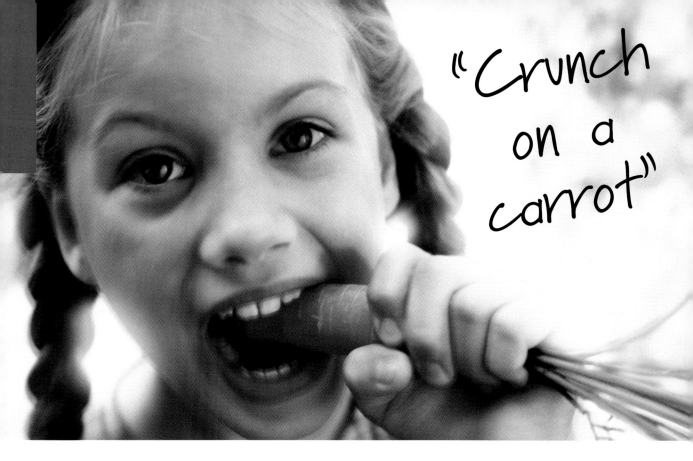

"Crunch on a carrot"

A healthy diet for children

Nutrition seems awash in numbers – percentages of this, milligrams of that. Fortunately, good nutrition still comes down to the basic food groups. A varied diet includes each one in the right amount.

The basic food groups

The Balance of Good Health is a pictorial guide in the shape of a plate showing the proportion and types of foods that are needed to make up a healthy balanced diet. The foods on the "Balanced Plate" are presented in these groups:

Carbohydrate foods (bread, potatoes, cereals, rice, and pasta): provide complex carbohydrates, fibre, vitamins, and some minerals.

Dairy foods (milk, yogurt, cheese, and other dairy foods): provide protein, vitamins, and minerals, especially calcium.

Protein foods (meat, fish, poultry, eggs, pulses, seeds, and nuts): provide protein as well as vitamins and minerals.

Fruits: provide fibre, vitamins, and minerals.

Vegetables: provide fibre, vitamins, and minerals.

Others (fats, oils, and sweets): provide little nutrient value. No single food contains all the essential nutrients the body needs to be healthy and function efficiently. The nutritional value of a person's diet depends on the overall mixture, or balance, of foods eaten over a period of time.

The Balance of Good Health does not apply to children under the age of two because they have high energy needs relative to their size. Between the ages of two and five, children can make a gradual transition to the recommended proportions. For young children and adolescents, the section of the plate allocated to dairy foods should be slightly bigger, reflecting their increased need for calcium.

Making sense of **servings and portions**

A balanced diet is one that is likely to include a large number or variety of foods from the different food groups (see previous page). Eating in this way helps to ensure that children – and parents – get an adequate intake of all the nutrients they need to remain healthy. To achieve the goal of a balanced diet, the Balance of Good Health suggests how many servings or portions of each of the food groups should be eaten every day. These servings are a standard size for everyone except for young children, who have smaller appetites (see page 95 for information about how much toddlers should eat).

GUIDELINES FOR DAILY SERVINGS

The Balance of Good Health recommends the number of servings of each food group that people should eat daily. As needs vary according to age, gender, and activity levels, a range of numbers is given. There are no specific recommendations for young children, but a good guide is to aim for the lowest number in each range.

FOOD GROUP	2- TO 6-YEAR-OLDS	OLDER THAN 6, INCLUDING ADULTS
Carbohydrate foods	at least 4 servings	6–11 servings
Dairy foods	2 servings	2–3 servings
Protein foods	2 servings	2–3 servings
Fruits	2–3 servings	2–4 servings
Vegetables	2–3 servings	3–5 servings
Others (fats, oils, sweets)	sparing use	sparing use

SIZING UP SERVINGS

Although standard servings are of a specified size, they vary depending on the type of food, even in the same food group (see below). These serving sizes are intended for adults; serving sizes for children may be smaller according to age and appetite. Note that juice can only be counted as one serving each day, however much you drink.

FOOD GROUP	STANDARD SERVING	SIZE COMPARISON (IF ANY)
Carbohydrate foods	1 slice of bread or toast	
	2 heaped tablespoons cooked rice	large ice cream scoop
	3 tablespoons breakfast cereal	
Dairy foods	200ml (7floz) milk	
	40g (1½ oz) cheese	matchbox
Protein foods	50–75g (2–3oz) cooked lean meat	pack of cards
	5 tablespoons cooked pulses	
	2 eggs	
	2 tablespoons peanut butter	ping pong ball
Fruits	1 medium whole fresh fruit such as an apple	tennis ball
	2 satsumas or kiwi fruit	
	1 heaped tablespoon dried fruit such as raisins	
Vegetables	3 tablespoons cooked vegetables such as peas	
	1 medium-sized mixed salad	cereal bowl
	150ml (5floz) vegetable (or fruit) juice	

Once-in-a-while foods

Eating can be an emotionally charged issue and certain foods can really get a parent annoyed, especially if you're trying to encourage healthy habits. But attempting to ban your child's favourite foods is unlikely to be successful.

Limiting snacks and treats

If your son has a soft spot for cheesy curls and he regularly overindulges, your impulse may be to forbid them. But it is wiser to allow him cheesy curls – as long as it's once in a while and in controlled portions. Snack foods have their place, but the trick is to limit them so they do not reduce your child's appetite for healthier fare.

The same goes for fast food, sweets, or other treats. Many snack and fast foods are high in calories and fat, particularly saturated fat, and low in nutrients. A typical deep-fried chicken nugget may contain as much as 50 percent fat, which is more than a regular fast-food burger.

Another way to deal with snacking is to offer alternatives that are just as appealing but more nutritious. Here are some delicious substitutes to try:

- Instead of a packet of crisps, try air-popped popcorn sprinkled with Parmesan cheese.
- Instead of ice cream, try fruit juice frozen into ice lollies.
- Instead of sweets, try apple or orange slices dipped into vanilla or fruit-flavoured yogurt.

Dilution is another smart strategy for parents. If your child likes crisps, occasionally buy a small quantity and use them in a snack mix that contains mostly healthier foods, such as popcorn, pretzels, and peanuts. If your child yearns for a sugary cereal, let him or her mix a small amount into a lower-sugar cereal as a compromise.

Also keep an eye on what's in your child's glass. Avoid sugary, fizzy drinks or offer them only very occasionally. Dilution works with drinks too, so mix fruit juice with water to reduce the calories. More often, serve your children milk or water to drink instead.

How much is enough?

Many parents wonder if their children get what they need for good health when their eating patterns seem erratic or fussy. Keeping a food log will help you understand your child's eating habits. If you record the type of food and amount your child eats for meals and snacks throughout each day over the course of a week, you will be able to make an accurate assessment of his or her diet.

Paying attention to the amount of food your child eats and when, as well as understanding serving sizes, may help you when assessing your child's diet. (For information on guidelines for daily servings and serving sizes, see page 41.) You may find that, more often than not, your child is eating in a healthy, well-balanced way.

What's in their **favourites?**

Most kids, particularly teenagers, love fast food, snacks, and sweetened drinks. But most of their favourite treats offer only "empty" calories (without many nutrients) – and plenty of those calories. These snacks and fast foods are also a source of unhealthy amounts of fats, sugar, and salt, so it's worth trying to limit them in your child's diet.

FOOD	CALORIES	TOTAL FAT/SATURATED FAT	SUGAR	SODIUM
Ice cream (1 scoop, 60g/2¼oz)	107	5g/3g	11g	37mg
Regular cola (1 can, 330ml/12floz)	129	0g	35g	26mg
Crisps (30g/1oz)	164	11g/3g	0g	321mg
Chocolate (1 small bar, 50g/2oz)	265	15g/9g	22g	60mg
Pizza (1 large slice, 100g/3½oz)	235	12g/6g	0g	570mg
Chicken nuggets (6 pieces)	300	18g/4g	0g	530mg

Once you know what your child is eating, you can analyze it in several different ways:

- total calorie intake;
- nutritional requirements, including carbohydrates, protein, fat, and fibre;
- number of servings of fruits, vegetables, and other important food groups.

You also can use the food log to look for other patterns, such as variety in food choices, number of meals and snacks eaten each day, and possible excesses such as too many empty-calorie snacks or drinks. Nutritional requirements vary by age. To check those for your child, see the appropriate age-specific chapter.

Working on the food log also will help your child see what he or she is eating and how this compares to the actual daily requirements. Depending on their age, kids can "score" themselves. To provide even more incentive, you might consider awarding stars on the chart for achieving specific goals, such as eating the minimum number of servings of food from the carbohydrate or dairy group every day or trying a new food. Your food log can be as simple as hand-written comments in a small notebook or as elaborate as a colour-coded chart studded with special stickers.

Five-a-day fruit and veg

Children in Britain eat on average only two servings of fruits and vegetables a day, and one in five eats no fruit at all. These children miss out on important nutrients as well as another component of a healthy diet: fibre. If you monitor what your child eats for a week or so, you may realize that one or two additional pieces of fruit and a few more servings of vegetables every day are in order. It's very important that children are given some fruits and vegetables at each meal. Once kids can count up to five they can start tracking their own progress towards the five-a-day goal.

Five-a-day may sound like a lot, especially if your family doesn't eat many fruits and vegetables, but servings can be small – children often find a huge pile of vegetables off-putting. It's much better to give an amount you know they will eat and gradually increase the portion size as they get older and their appetites grow.

Should kids eat a low-fat diet?

Restrictive diets aren't recommended for children and fat, despite the bad press, is not The Enemy. In fact, for young children, fat and cholesterol play important roles in brain development. For children younger than two, fat intake should not be restricted and they should be given full-fat milk. Starting at age two, children should eat a varied diet with 30–35 percent of calories from fat (if they have a healthy appetite they can switch to semi-skimmed milk).

It's true that most kids eat too much fat, so here are some ways to keep your child's fat intake at 30–35 percent.

- Offer naturally low-fat foods, such as fruits and vegetables, whole grains, and lean meats, as well as low-fat dairy products.
- When cooking meat, opt for grilling or roasting (on a rack). These methods allow fat to drip away during cooking, cutting down on calories too. Frying keeps food in its own fat or requires added fat.
- Resist low-fat biscuits and other snacks. They may be high in calories and are easy to overeat.

tips

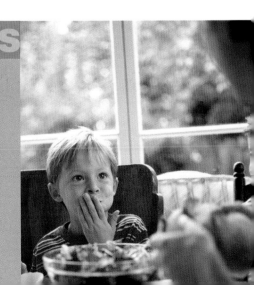

How to be a role model

- Make time for your meals, even if it's just 15 minutes for a sandwich and a piece of fruit.
- Sit down to eat – it doesn't take much more time.
- Put your work or book away and concentrate on your meal. You'll be able to return to your project soon enough, with renewed energy from a healthy meal.

- Choose a nutritious snack, such as yogurt with a few flaked almonds or other nuts sprinkled on top.
- Don't skip meals.
- Don't eat on the move, such as in the car rushing off somewhere.
- Don't eat quickly while standing at the refrigerator.
- Don't "graze" or snack all day instead of eating meals.

How to help kids eat healthier

It's all well and good to know what your child should eat, but getting the food from the plate to the stomach can be a challenge. It may seem wrong, but letting kids have some control is the way to go.

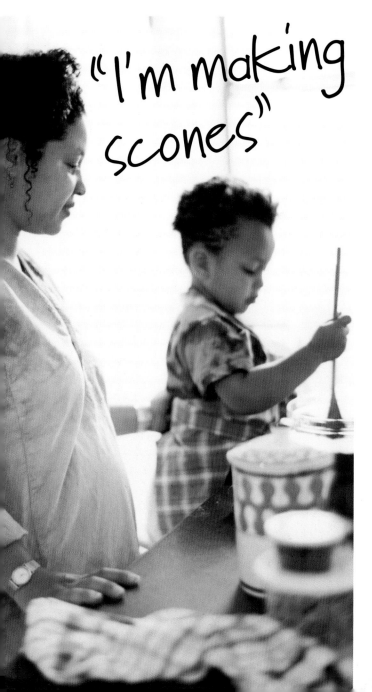

"I'm making scones"

No prodding or pleading

Nutritionists now put forth a simple rule for parents: you decide what foods are available and the child decides what to eat and even whether to eat at all. Yes, this means they can walk away from the table. But because you control the food, it also means that they won't have the option of opening a packet of crisps and using snacks to fill the void.

Giving children this kind of control might go against the parental grain. We may want efficient eating and clean plates, but this is not how kids operate. And that's actually a good thing. Children, especially younger ones, respond to their own hunger cues. If you can respect those cues too, your child may be on the way to a healthy and pleasurable relationship with food.

The challenge of fussy eaters

Some children may become so fussy that they refuse to eat anything but, say, cheese sandwiches for weeks on end. This is obviously not ideal, but the parent who responds by forcing the child to eat other foods won't solve the problem. A better course is to continue offering a range of foods and hope that this phase will pass, which it inevitably does.

When trying to introduce healthy foods to infants and fussy toddlers, don't give up too easily. It could take as many as ten tries before a child accepts a new food. Keep offering, without forcing, and your child may end up liking it after all.

Sometimes what seems like fussiness is actually just preference, so it pays to know what your child likes and dislikes. Just like you, they're going to favour some kinds of foods. One nine-year-old girl, to her mother's dismay, refused to eat breakfast, heading into her school day with an empty tummy. But after talking it over, it turned out that it wasn't breakfast that the girl disliked. It was the kinds of foods that her mother offered – typical fare including toast and muesli. The girl preferred smooth textures in the morning, such as yogurt. Problem solved.

It's true, however, that parents may face disappointment when they set out to instil healthy eating habits. Children like what they like and sometimes no amount of choices or vegetables cut into fancy shapes can change that. If this is the case, try not to dig in your heels as that can make mealtimes tense instead of relaxed and enjoyable.

Have a realistic attitude

Food can become linked to negative feelings early on. If parents repeatedly grow frustrated when introducing an infant or young child to new foods, the child picks up on the mood. And if parents use dessert as a reward, the sweet treat can become the goal, making supper just something to get through on the way there. These practices can create unhealthy eating patterns instead of resolving them.

Anyone who's ever fed an infant knows that food and comfort are intrinsically linked, and that food can be a way to show love and care. But be wary of using food to praise or reward a child, punish a child, soothe hurt feelings, or as the sole expression of love. Consistently using food in this way can build a dependence on food for support or even happiness. Having a child skip a meal as a punishment can tie food to disapproval. Once such connections have been forged, they can last a lifetime.

Children also pick up on adults' attitudes about food, so be aware of your approaches to eating too. Don't expect a child to want to try a variety of foods if you regularly eat cottage cheese for supper. If you view food as a collection of unwanted calories, your child may adopt a similar outlook. Instead, turn mealtimes into pleasurable, social events. Use them to your advantage by:

- eating together as a family;
- offering a selection of fruits and vegetables;
- modelling good habits by eating healthy foods;
- encouraging small, "try it" portions of a tablespoon or two;
- turning off the TV while you eat.

Kids in the kitchen

Try turning the tables and get your child involved in the selection of menus and the preparation of meals. This will do more than just expand your child's repertoire as far as eating. A child who's at home in the kitchen feels empowered about food and gains first-hand knowledge of nutrition. This lays the groundwork for making healthy food choices later on.

If children are very young, give them small pans, spoons, and other safe utensils so they can pretend to cook along with you. For younger school-age kids, let them prepare recipes involving five or fewer ingredients and where everything is mixed and cooked in the same container. If your child can read, let him or her read out the recipe – a great way to practise reading skills. Older kids can take over the creation of a meal if they're interested. Let them be completely in charge of dinner occasionally, from selecting recipes and shopping with you for ingredients to cooking and serving.

tips

Children and food: 10 tips for parents

1 Parents control the supply lines: You decide which foods to buy and when to serve them.

2 Kids decide if and what to eat: From the foods you offer, they get to choose what they eat or whether to eat at all.

3 Forget the "clean plate" goal: Let your children stop eating when they feel they've had enough.

4 Start them young: Food preferences are developed early in life, so offer a variety of foods.

5 Rewrite the kids' menu: Who says children only want to eat hamburgers, sausages, macaroni cheese, and

pizza? Let your children try new foods and they might surprise you with their willingness to experiment.

6 Drink calories count: Cola and other sweetened drinks add extra calories and get in the way of good nutrition.

7 Put sweets in their place: Occasional sweets are fine, but don't turn dessert into the main reason for eating dinner.

8 Food is not love: Find better ways to say I love you.

9 Children do as you do: Be a role model and eat healthily yourself.

10 Turn off the TV: You'll also turn off the advertising and mindless snacking.

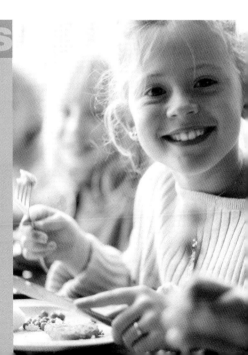

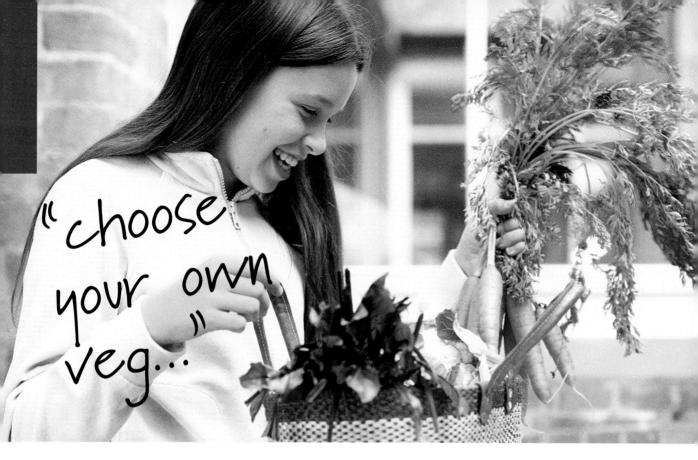

"choose your own veg..."

Be an informed food shopper

Learning to shop wisely will help you put the best foods on your family's table. Find out what to look for at the shop or supermarket, whether you're buying fresh, frozen, or canned products.

When fresh is best

It's no surprise that fine restaurants use the freshest fruits and vegetables. Their appearance and taste speak for themselves. But it can be challenging to buy and serve fresh produce. For a start, it's not always easy to find and it can be expensive. Also, it can easily spoil before you get a chance to eat it. The secrets lie in knowing where to shop, how to choose excellent produce, and how to store it until you're ready to serve it.

Choose shops that feature fresh produce and turn over their stocks regularly. It's also worth trying farmers' markets and farm shops to see what's available locally. Wherever you choose to shop, it pays to know the time of year that your

favourite fruits and vegetables are in season. Buying in-season produce is often a bargain, but don't buy more than you can store or use before it spoils. A good way to teach your children about seasonal fruit is by visiting a pick-your-own farm so they can pick the fresh fruit themselves.

When you don't pick it off the vine or plant yourself, how do you know produce is fresh? Whether it's melon or runner beans, all fruits and vegetables give hints about their ripeness and freshness.

- Choose vegetables that look fresh and colourful. Most should be crisp and firm: with vegetables such as runner or French beans, for example, don't buy them if they are limp or showing signs of decay.

myth: **Organic food is healthier than conventionally grown products.**

fact: The jury is still out on this question – while some studies show that organic fruit and vegetables do contain higher levels of vitamins and minerals, others show there is no significant difference. Organic foods are produced by growers or suppliers who emphasize environmental protection and resource conservation. In general, organic growers don't use most pesticides, synthetic fertilizer, or other processes such as irradiation. With animal products, antibiotics are not given routinely as preventatives against disease or as growth promoters.

Organic products are typically more expensive than those produced by non-organic methods, but are attractive to consumers seeking the most natural foods available. And organic produce that is grown locally will reach the supermarket at its freshest. However, much organic produce is imported into the UK. It may come from countries where regulations are not as strict as those in the UK, so be sure to check where the produce originated.

- When choosing fruits, avoid bruised pieces, but remember that a perfect exterior doesn't necessarily mean the best quality: if it's melon you're after, for example, the best will have a yellowish cast and may be misshapen, but it will smell pleasantly sweet.

Careful storage will help you ensure that fresh produce lasts longer. Keep most fruits and vegetables in the refrigerator at a temperature of 5°C (40°F). Vegetables will keep in the refrigerator for two to five days; root vegetables such as carrots will keep even longer. Store potatoes and onions in a cool, dark place for maximum freshness.

The merits of frozen and canned

For convenience you can't beat frozen and canned fruits and vegetables, the best of which rival fresh when it comes to taste and nutrition. Used in a recipe, your family may not be able to tell the difference between fresh and frozen fruit and vegetables or those from a can. A recent study of 1500 people found that dishes prepared with canned ingredients were just as appealing as those that contained fresh or frozen produce.

Whether fresh or frozen, you'll want to check the label to see what you're buying. Some frozen vegetables, for instance, are packaged with extra salt and fat. Instead, choose products that are packaged without any sauces or additives. With canned fruits, look for varieties that pack the fruit in juice, not syrup.

- Don't buy a package of frozen vegetables if the bag is ripped or the box is soggy or torn.
- With canned products, watch out for any can that has a large dent or a swollen appearance, or one from which some of the juices are leaking out.

When you bring cans of food home, store them at a temperature of no more than 24°C (75°F). They will keep their quality for about a year. If there isn't a best before date on a can, it's a good idea to label it with the date of purchase. Frozen food will keep best if stored in a freezer that stays at -18°C (0°F).

Other convenience foods

If you often have to prepare quick meals, you may rely on the convenient short-cuts that are readily available in the supermarket aisles. Flavoured risotto in a box, spaghetti in a can, and frozen ready-meals fall into this category, as do pre-seasoned raw chicken breasts and pre-boxed lunches for kids. There's such a range of convenience foods that consumers need to consider what each one has to offer. It's worth taking the time to look carefully at the cost of the food and its convenience, as well as its nutritional value, before making a decision about whether or not to buy it.

Often convenience foods are more expensive than cooking a meal from scratch. And, unlike cooking from scratch, the cook has little or no control over how the dish is made or what's in it. Sometimes, of course, the fact that it is quick and easy makes it worth its price. Just be sure that it has something to offer in terms of nutrition.

Try to avoid convenience foods that are high in sugar or fat, particularly saturated or trans fats. A quick scan of the ingredients list can be very telling. Think twice about buying foods if any of the following ingredients appear as one of the top three in the list: fructose, honey, glucose, dextrose, maltose, sucrose, corn syrup (all of which are types of sugar), sugar, hydrogenated vegetable oil, coconut oil, lard, palm kernel oil, beef tallow, or shortening.

Reading labels

Labels on bags, packets, bottles, and cans of food are there to help you decide how a food can fit into your family's diet. Find out how to scan these labels for the information you need, whether you're buying frozen peas or digestive biscuits.

Look for the label

Over the past few years, food labels have been growing increasingly comprehensive. At one time you might have been lucky to learn what was in the packet you were buying, but today labelling is helpful and easy to read, to protect consumers. For example, if a food contains more than one ingredient, a complete list of the ingredients is required. Manufacturers also must give a breakdown of the nutrient content so consumers can compare similar products and choose foods according to their individual dietary needs. Labels must also state how long the food can be kept and how to store it; how to prepare and cook it; the name and address of the maker, packer, or seller of the food; and sometimes the place of origin. There's a lot of information in that panel. Here are some of the most important lines to check, when deciding whether to buy something or not.

Portion size and portions per container: You'll find out how large a normal portion or serving size is and how many portions are in that packet. Pay attention to portion size because it's common to eat more than one portion.

Typical or average values: These can be tricky when it comes to children because they are given for 100g or 100ml of the food (and sometimes also per average portion or serving). So the amounts may not be on target for children. However, you can still use this information to determine if something is a rich or poor source of nutrients. For instance, a food supplying only 1g of fibre cannot be considered a source of fibre, either for an adult or a child.

Energy content: This line will tell you the number of kcals (kilocalories) there are in 100g or 100ml of the food (See page 33 for an explanation of kilocalories.) A kilojoule (kj) is another way to measure energy: 1 kcal = 4.2 kj.

Fat: This will tell you how many grams of fat are in 100g or 100ml of the food. Look for the breakdown showing how much of the total fat content is saturated, which is the type of fat known to raise blood cholesterol levels and be a risk factor for heart disease.

Sodium: This shows how many grams of sodium are in 100g or 100ml of the food. A gram of sodium is equal to 2.5g of salt. (See page 38 for recommended daily intake.)

Carbohydrate: This gives the total carbohydrate content of 100g or 100ml of the food, as well as how many grams of the carbohydrate come from sugars.

Fibre: This will tell you how much fibre is in 100g or 100ml of the food (3g or more makes the food a source of fibre).

Protein: This is the gram weight of protein in 100g or 100ml of the food.

Additional information: A label may show if the food is suitable for people with dietary restrictions, such as "Suitable for vegetarians" or "This product contains nuts".

NUTRITION INFORMATION

Typical values per 100g		Portion
Energy	1741kJ	1219kJ
	414kcal	290kcal
Protein	3.5g	2.5g
Carbohydrate	65.8g	46.1g
of which sugars	49.1g	14.4g
Fat	15.2g	10.6g
of which saturates	3.6g	2.5g
Fibre	2.3g	1.6g
Sodium	0.1g	0.1g
Based on 8 portions per cake		

INGREDIENTS:
Raisins, glacé cherries, wheatflour, egg, partially hydrogenated vegetable oil, pecan nuts, sugar, glucose syrup, honey, flavourings, emulsifiers (E471, E435), spices, salt, preservative (E202), gelling agent (E440), acidity regulator (E330), colours (E127, E133, E102, E129)

- THIS PRODUCT CONTAINS NUTS
- SUITABLE FOR VEGETARIANS

Typical or average values These can help you determine if the food is a good or poor source of certain nutrients.

Protein The protein content must be shown, even when there is very little or none.

Sugars This is a good line to check, but it will not distinguish between added sugar and naturally occurring sugars.

Fat The fat content is broken down to show how much of it is saturated.

Ingredients All ingredients must be listed in descending order of weight. Additives and preservatives are often shown by their E (European) numbers.

Trans fats If hydrogenated or partially hydrogenated oil is listed in the ingredients, trans fats will be present. (For an explanation of trans fats, see page 36.)

Label lingo
It's worth the effort it takes to become a savvy label-reader so you can assess a food's nutritional value.

Storing and preparing food

Providing nutritious meals for your family goes well beyond buying the food. Those who prepare food need to know the basics about kitchen hygiene and how to prevent food-borne illnesses. Uncooked foods – even cake mixture – should be off-limits for children.

Good kitchen practice

- Check the temperature of your refrigerator to ensure that it is 5°C (40°F) and your freezer is -18°C (0°F) or less. Cool temperatures keep bacteria in foods from multiplying.
- Don't keep or buy fruit with broken skin because the opening creates an avenue for bacteria.
- Keep raw fish, meat, and poultry and their juices away from other foods in the refrigerator and on work surfaces. Store meat and poultry in the bottom of the fridge.
- Wash hands, cutting boards, and knives or other utensils thoroughly after preparing raw foods, especially meats and eggs. Wash cutting boards separately from other dishes and utensils.
- Use separate utensils and plates for cooking and serving meat, poultry, fish, or eggs (or wash the utensils in hot, soapy water before using them to serve).
- Cook meats thoroughly, using a meat thermometer to check. Minced beef, especially, must be cooked until it is brown inside, not red or pink.
- Refrigerate any leftovers as soon as possible after cooking. If left at room temperature, bacteria that may be in the food will multiply quickly.
- Scrub all fruits and vegetables with water to remove any pesticide residue, bacteria, and dirt.
- Some foods (such as home-made ice cream, mayonnaise, and chocolate mousse) may contain raw eggs or unspecified raw food products and could be contaminated with salmonella, so they should not be given to children. Find out whether raw eggs are used and, if so, avoid them. Unpasteurized milk and milk products and unpasteurized apple juice also could cause food-borne illness.
- Children whose immunity is weakened by diseases such as cancer or AIDS should avoid uncooked foods that could carry listeriosis bacteria. These include soft cheeses like feta, Brie, and Camembert, and blue-veined cheeses. Ready-cooked meats from the delicatessen must be cooked again before serving to kill any bacteria.

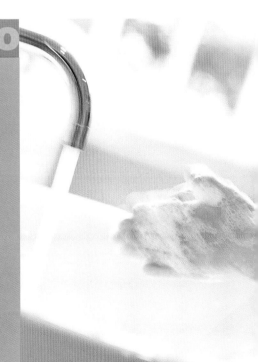

info

Teaching kids about kitchen safety

Any time you have children in the kitchen, you'll need to think about safety issues. Younger children should be closely supervised, so they don't burn or cut themselves. But there are plenty of safe tasks they will enjoy. Here are some ideas:
- washing vegetables
- mixing pancake batter
- sprinkling on spices and herbs.

In between tasks, let them lay the table, take everyone's drink order, or pretend to cook alongside you.

Care needs to be taken with older children too, as they may be overconfident of their abilities. Ensure that you:
- monitor their use of cookers, ovens, and other kitchen appliances;
- teach them the proper way to use knives and other sharp kitchen tools.

But don't let your safety concerns make them feel unwelcome in the kitchen. Invite your children to pick new dishes to try and encourage them to make their lunches.

Good hygiene

Kids also need to learn about another kind of kitchen safety – preventing food-borne illnesses, such as E coli, salmonellosis, campylobacter infections, and listeriosis (see above). Even the youngest child can learn to wash hands before getting involved in a cooking project. As kids get older you can educate them about proper food storage, preparation, and cleaning up.

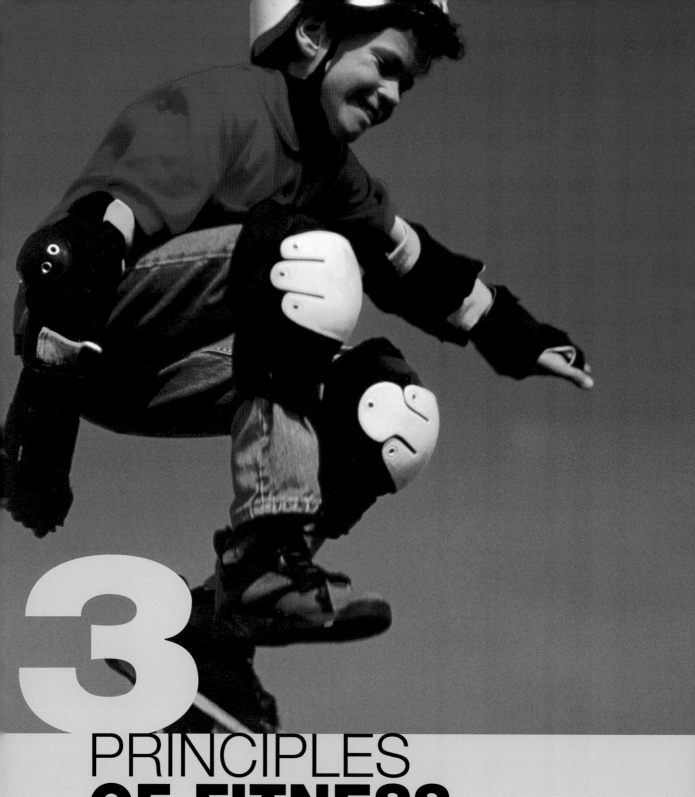

3

PRINCIPLES
OF FITNESS

Most young children are **naturally physically active** and love to move around. But **older kids may slow down**. Fight the couch potato trend and **help your child** cultivate a love of activity that will last a lifetime.

Fit and healthy for life

To many people, "fitness" is something that requires hours in the gym. But fitness can simply mean being healthy and having a body that's strong enough to do everything you want and need it to do.

A love of physical activity

Nearly all children start out fit and eager to be active. Just consider the unstoppable force that is the average pre-school child, who runs, spins, leaps, and climbs at every opportunity. But as children get older, they start to encounter obstacles that may make it difficult to be active. There are plenty of explanations:

- the increasing demands of school;
- a feeling among some kids that they aren't good at sports;
- concerns about safety that prevent children from having the freedom to roam their own neighbourhoods.

Despite these barriers, parents can help their children develop a love of physical activity at a young age, which, if encouraged, can be carried with them throughout their lives.

The many benefits of exercise

There are a great many health benefits for children who are physically active. A child who is active will:

- have stronger muscles and stronger bones;
- have a leaner body because exercise helps control body fat;
- be less likely to become overweight;
- decrease the risk of developing Type 2 diabetes;
- possibly lower blood pressure and blood cholesterol levels;
- have a better outlook on life.

Regular exercise also strengthens the heart muscle, which improves its effectiveness. A stronger heart pumps more blood with each beat, which means it is able to deliver oxygen throughout the body more efficiently.

All children can be physically fit

For the more athletic child, physical training can improve performance so the child may be able to run faster, jump higher, or throw a ball farther. But fitness is not an exclusive

"boing! boing! boing!"

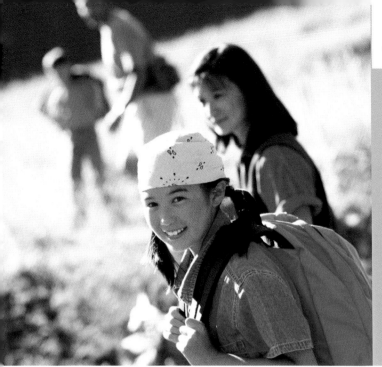

What parents say...
about exercise

"I have a boy who is five and a girl seven. What I've learned is that they must not view what we're doing as 'exercise'. My wife and I enjoy going on walks, but the children hate it. Even if we allow them to take their bikes or rollerblades it's still a bore – it's not what they would choose to do. So I set aside four or five hours every Saturday or Sunday when I allow them to pick the activity, be it swimming, cycling, rock climbing, or playing tag. But it must be something that I consider exercise (of course I don't tell them that). One day my daughter asked why we do this every week. I explained that it's important for everyone to get exercise. Her reply wasn't what I expected, but was what I wanted. She said, 'But we don't exercise, we just play'."

club limited only to the child who is gifted at sport or who has an athletic body type. All children can be physically fit, whatever their abilities and interests. Parents can influence their child's fitness habits – positively or negatively. A child who has active parents is six times more likely to be physically active. And it's not just what you do and say about exercise, but the way you deliver the message. Don't let your child view physical activity as a burden or another boring task. Help your child see exercise as a broad category that includes a wide range of physical activities to choose from.

As the parent, it's your job to help your child discover which activities or sports he or she most enjoys. Then try to find ways for your child to participate in them. This can sometimes be problematic, as a recent study showed. In the survey, parents of nine- to 13-year-olds acknowledged the following obstacles to getting their kids physically fit:

- expense
- transportation problems
- parents' lack of time
- lack of opportunities in the area
- lack of neighbourhood safety.

Expense and transportation problems were considered the top two issues. These problems were most acute in lower-income households, but also mentioned by middle- and upper-income parents. It's true that sports participation can be expensive, but it's also true that low-cost alternatives are

often available. To get your child involved at little or no expense, contact your child's school, the local authority sports and leisure department, community centre, and organizations such as the YMCA.

If transportation is a problem, look for after-school programmes to alleviate one leg of the journey. Also consider sharing the transportation of children with other parents and, when a child is old enough, whether public transport is an option.

But, most importantly, teach your child that physical activity doesn't have to come as part of an organized sport or programme. Lead an active lifestyle together, doing errands on foot instead of by car and spending free time at the park. Also invest in balls and skipping ropes.

Of 3800 children surveyed in a recent study, 77 percent said they had participated in free-play physical activity during the previous week, while only about 39 percent said they had participated in an organized physical activity like a team sport. A mix of both types of activity is ideal, especially as a child reaches school age. Being part of a team is a way to make friends and teaches a child about teamwork and following rules. The balance between free play and organized activities is your decision and your child's, but make sure your child gets enough regular physical activity. (For specific recommendations, see page 54.) If your child took part in this survey, what would he or she have said?

Why children need physical activity

Children need to be fit for the same reasons adults do: to improve their health and ensure that they can perform normal daily tasks and activities. People who are fit sleep better and are better able to handle the challenges that a typical day presents.

Developing skills and fitness

Regular exercise helps children to grow, to build strong muscles and bones, and to develop important motor skills. We understand this with babies and toddlers as they learn to sit up, walk, and then to run, but regular exercise remains important as children get older.

Even the older child who seems very capable is learning new skills, and regular physical activity helps strengthen his or her developing body. Repetition leads to mastery of the basic skills, from throwing and catching and skipping to more precise movements, such as turning a pirouette in ballet or deftly placing a shot in tennis.

Depending on their age and development, children need different amounts of activity and types of exercise. For example, young children (aged one to five years) shouldn't be inactive for more than 60 minutes unless they're sleeping. Children up to the age of 12 should get at least 60 minutes of free-play time every day.

Babies and toddlers get much of the activity they need through interaction and play with their parents. As children get older, their readiness to participate in different types of physical activity depends on age, development, and individual likes and dislikes. At any age, there's no point forcing a child to play a sport if it's not fun for them.

How much is **enough?**

AGE	DEVELOPMENT	DAILY ACTIVITY	SUGGESTED ACTIVITIES	WHAT PARENTS SHOULD DO
Infant	learning to roll over, sit, stand, walk	no specific recommendations	physical activity should encourage motor development; no formal programme necessary	provide a safe play space; avoid walkers; limit time in car seats, pushchairs, buggies
Toddler (1–3 years)	walking, running, climbing, kicking, jumping	1½ hours	play (especially outdoors), smaller scale playground equipment, push-and-pull toys, ride-on vehicles, balls	ensure 30 minutes structured activity daily with games, plus at least 60 minutes of unstructured play time
Pre-school (3–5 years)	hopping, balancing on one foot, throwing and catching, pedalling, skipping	1½–2 hours	catch, tag, playground time, trikes and bikes, bat and balls, tumbling and dance	provide 30–60 minutes of structured activity daily, plus at least 60 minutes of unstructured play time
School-age (6–12 years)	building more complex movements; developing hand-eye coordination; starting to understand rules	1½–2 hours	skipping rope, swimming, cycling, team sports (non-competitive during earlier years), outdoor play	provide home play equipment; be sure children get 30–60 minutes physical activity daily, as well as at least 60 minutes unstructured play time
Adolescent (13 and older)	body changes in puberty, growing taller and stronger	30–60 minutes	choose according to interests and age – competitive sports, classes, jogging, swimming, cycling	provide equipment and/or transportation; ensure at least three 20-minute sessions of more vigorous exercise weekly

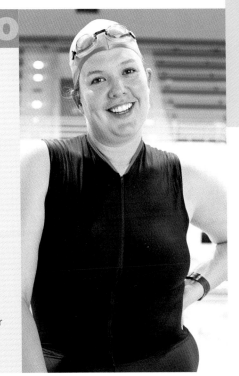

info

Motivating overweight kids

Exercise offers tremendous benefits for overweight children, but it may be hard for many of them to get started. Be sensitive to reasons why an overweight child may not want to exercise, such as embarrassment over wearing a swimsuit or shorts or changing in front of other kids before PE class.

- Find activities that interest your child – some suit overweight children better than others. For example, swimming and walking are ideal choices because they are easier on the joints.
- If your child is more comfortable exercising at home, try an age-appropriate exercise video. Older children may be interested in using home gym equipment, such as a treadmill or stationary bike.

- Let them shop for workout clothes and trainers that they like wearing and that offer adequate support. Overweight children may be in poor physical condition, but as long as your GP approves encourage them to get moving. Your child can start by walking five minutes a day and add a minute each day until they reach the exercise goal of at least 30 minutes every day.

An overweight child who has little experience with exercise is at risk of injury. Teach your child to warm up, and cool down afterwards. Overweight kids are at increased risk of dehydration too, so be sure they drink plenty of water.

Never criticize your child for being inactive, but be sure to praise him or her for making efforts to get moving. Also offer to exercise with your child.

Pre-school children don't have the skills that older kids have mastered, such as throwing and running at the same time. But a child as young as four or five may enjoy learning basic skills through tumbling, a dance class, or learning to throw a ball in the park. Pre-teens and teenagers can be left more in charge of choosing the kind of exercise they want to do – as long as they get enough. So find out what your child's interests are and work together to help him or her get enough physical activity. (For information about how to choose an activity that suits your child, see page 137.)

Organized sports

You may wonder when your child can start organized sports. Although some programmes are designed for younger kids, six is a good age for most – any class or club for children younger than this should stress development of basic skills and having fun. By six or seven, though, children are more physically ready, they have a longer attention span, and they can begin to grasp simple rules.

As children get older, they can start to handle more responsibility, such as keeping score and keeping track of wins and losses for their team. But be cautious about teams that require try-outs, many hours of practice, and a lot of travelling, or that emphasize winning. While some children are motivated by competitive play, the average child may not be ready for the increased pressure until he or she is 11 or 12 years old. Remember, too, that even with the more competitive teams, the atmosphere should remain positive and supportive for all the participants.

Free play

In addition to sport, parents should encourage free play. Unlike organized activities, such as gymnastics or playing football or rugby, free play allows your child to choose how to be active.

- For younger children, free play might include imaginative play, action songs such as "Simon Says" and "Hokey Cokey", or dancing.
- As children get older, hopscotch, tag, or "piggy in the middle" may be more fun.
- Free play for pre-teens and teenagers might mean skateboarding, rollerblading, or cycling.

(For more advice on activities for different age groups, see the age-specific chapters.)

How to get physically fit

Though heredity and home environment affect a child's ability to get fit, almost all children – and adults – can enjoy the sense of well-being that comes with regular physical activity.

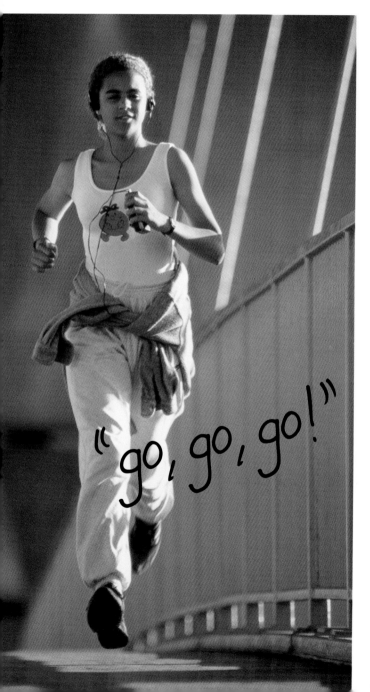

"go, go, go!"

What is fitness?

Physical activity is any movement of the large muscles of the body that results in burning more calories (see page 33) than would be used while resting. Physical fitness can be achieved through regular physical activity.

Fitness can be divided into two types: health-related and performance or skill-related. Health-related fitness improves heart and muscle function, strengthens bones, and increases well-being. An active child is more likely to be active into adulthood when health-related fitness has important long-term benefits. These benefits include improved quality of life and a reduced risk of developing certain diseases, such as Type 2 diabetes and heart disease.

Performance fitness includes improvement in speed, balance, agility, and coordination – the types of activities that help people excel at sports. Some children may focus on improving performance just because they like the tangible results of being faster, stronger, or more capable. Usually, while focusing on gains in performance fitness, children are helping themselves achieve health-related fitness as well.

The three elements

If you've ever watched children in a playground, you know that they love to move their bodies, whether it's climbing to the top of the slide or swinging from the monkey bars. Without thinking about it, they are developing the three elements of fitness: endurance, strength, and flexibility. While different kids will have different abilities, all children should regularly be doing activities that involve all three elements.

Endurance is developed when you move your body in a way that increases your heart rate and quickens your breathing in a sustained way. Described as aerobic exercise ("with air"), this improves the body's ability to deliver oxygen to all its cells, thus increasing the aerobic capacity and, with it, endurance. Kids get this kind of exercise when they run or jog, skip, jump, and play.

Exercises **for flexibility**

Body flexibility comes in handy all the time, even when you're doing something as simple as tying your shoelaces. Being flexible means that your muscles and joints stretch and bend easily, so your limbs can move through their full range of motion. With activities such as practising a split or touching their toes, or stretching exercises like these, children develop flexibility.

Sit and twist
Start with legs straight. Bend left leg and cross it over right leg so left foot is alongside right knee. Bring right arm across body and hold outer side of left leg near knee. Slowly twist body and look over left shoulder. Hold stretch for 10–30 seconds. Repeat on other side.

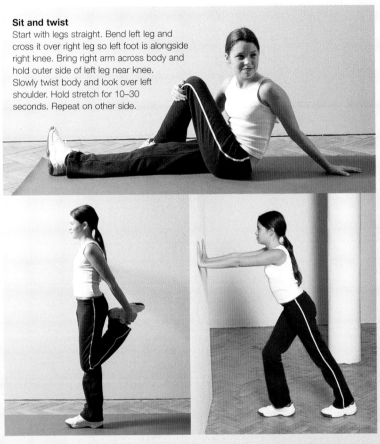

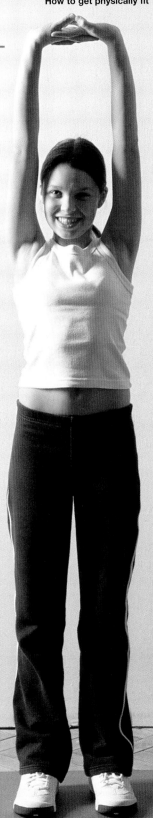

Thigh stretch
Standing up straight, bend one knee and bring ankle up behind body. Grasp ankle firmly in hand on same side. Keep bent leg beside other leg. Pull ankle up until you feel tension in front of thigh. Hold this for 15–20 seconds. Repeat twice for each leg.

Calf stretch
Place hands flat against wall with arms and back straight. Bend one knee slightly and extend other leg backwards, keeping foot flat on floor. You should feel tension in back of extended leg. Hold this stretch for 15–20 seconds. Repeat twice with each leg.

Overhead stretch
Clasp hands together and raise them, palms upwards, above head, stretching your arms. Hold stretch for 20 seconds.

Resistance band exercises **for strength**

Some people think that strength training means lifting weights to get big muscles. But strength training offers a range of benefits for children. They will have improved muscle tone and their muscles will better support their joints. Also weight-bearing exercise, such as running or jumping, builds stronger bones. (To find out more about weight training for children, see below.) Resistance bands, which are strong elastic tubes or bands, can be a safe alternative to free weights or weight machines. Start with a set of ten of the exercises below and add additional sets as your child's fitness level improves.

Pull out

Stand with feet shoulder width apart, shoulders down. Hold handles in front of chest, palms facing in. Inhale. Stretch band out, straight across in front of body, keeping elbows slightly bent. (Children under ten should start out pulling only halfway.) Exhale. Hold for two counts, then control band back to starting position. Repeat.

Rowing

Put one handle of band under arch of foot. With feet together, hold other handle with both hands, palms in. Inhale. Raise hands no higher than chin, lifting elbows to side. Exhale. Lower band slowly. Repeat.

Arm curl

Place one handle of band under arch of foot. Slightly separate feet. Inhale. Draw band up towards shoulder, keeping back straight and holding upper arm against body. Exhale. Lower band slowly. Repeat.

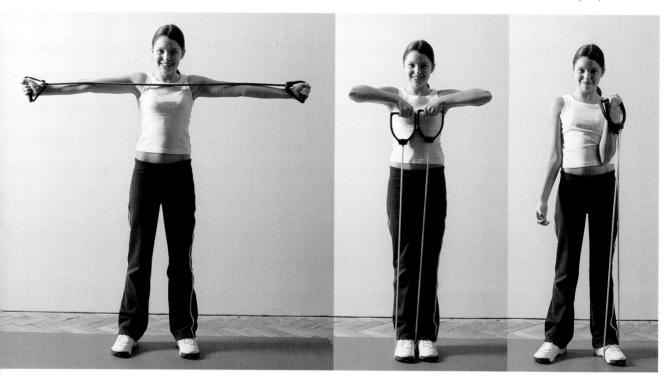

Q: Is weight training safe for my 12-year-old son?

A: Some boys at this age are interested in lifting weights because they want to build muscles, especially if they see their peers maturing. Strength training, under the right conditions, can increase muscle tone and may help your son feel better about his body, but it won't build muscle until he reaches puberty.

Talk to your GP about your son's interest in strength training. With the doctor's approval, seek out a certified athletic trainer or coach who has experience training children. That person can help your son start a safe and appropriate programme, ensuring that he won't be lifting heavy weights and will be supervised during the workout. Be sure your son uses light weights and does several repetitions.

Floor exercises **for strength**

If a muscle is strong, it can exert a lot of force. For instance, a strong arm can curl a heavy barbell. But children don't need to lift weights to be strong. The simplest way for children to improve muscle strength is to use their own body weight as resistance during strengthening exercises. Doing repetitions of these sorts of exercises builds both muscle strength and endurance. Of course, children also work on their muscles by crossing the monkey bars in the playground or learning to hold a handstand. Get your child to begin with a set of ten of each of the exercises below and add additional sets as his or her fitness improves.

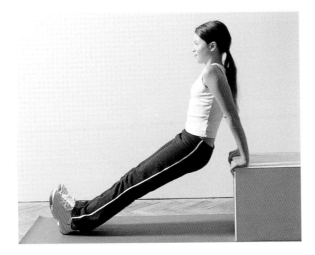

Press-up
Lie flat on floor, face down, hands under shoulders, fingers straight. Bend knees and bring feet up at 90° angle to body. Lift body off floor by straightening arms; keep back straight and knees bent. Lower body until you have a 90° angle at elbows. Repeat.

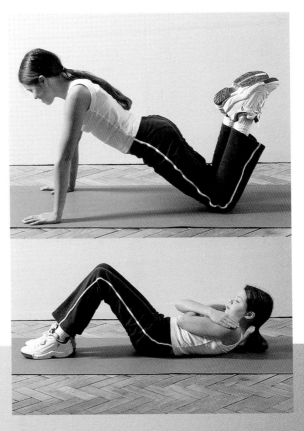

Seat drop
With back to heavy block or sturdy chair and straight arms kept a shoulder width apart, place hands on front edge of block or chair. Stretch out legs straight in front, feet together and heels on floor. Lower body until arms are bent 90°, then straighten arms to pull yourself up.

Curl-up
Lie on floor on back, legs bent and feet flat. Cross arms on chest. Lift chest towards knees until shoulders come off floor. Lie back down.

Leg lift
Lie on side with knee of bottom leg bent forward at 30–40° angle. Have ankle/foot of upper leg in a neutral position. Lift upper leg straight up to shoulder height. Hold for five seconds, then lower leg back down.

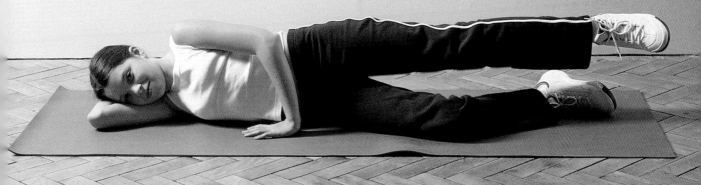

How to help children get fit

The best way for children to get physical activity is by incorporating regular exercise into their daily routine, whether it be involvement in organized sports or enjoying free play. It's an excellent fitness strategy for the whole family to adopt.

Motivating your child

This is the $64,000 question: what will motivate children and teenagers to get fit? The answers can be found in the positive experience of kids who are fit and who enjoy physical activity. These children feel they are good at whatever activity they're doing, they feel accepted by their peers and important adults, and – most importantly – they have fun.

Here's how those good feelings about activity are built:

- Children enjoy activity because it's fun.
- Because they're active, they improve their skills.
- Because their skills improve, they get praise from peers, parents, and adults.
- Because of that praise, they gain self-confidence.
- And as a result, they enjoy physical activity even more.

Though it may be easiest with a child who's naturally interested in sports and athletically gifted, any child can be motivated. Start by finding something your child enjoys doing or is interested in. Then be sure the coaching staff or teacher is trained and knows the importance of praise and support. As a parent, you should also be supportive about the child's performance, while at the same time keeping expectations realistic. The goal is to help your child feel that he or she is succeeding.

You'll want to keep your child's age in mind because children need different kinds of positive reinforcement as they grow from babies to teenagers. Infants and toddlers need attention, stimulation, and encouragement. School-age children feel competent when they master simple tasks, try

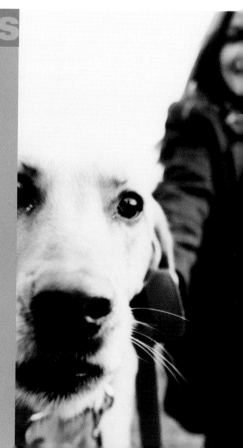

tips

Getting children to commit

Here are some good ways to work with your child and encourage a commitment to regular physical activity.

Create an activity menu Younger children especially will enjoy making an activity menu and using the menu options to plan a calendar of activities. Work with your child to draw up a list of favourite activities. Put this list where your child can see it and refer to it often. You can then let your child use the activity menu to create a calendar of planned activities. It also might be a good source of ideas for those moments when your child says, "I'm bored".

- Everyday activities: walking the dog, helping tidy the house, and walking to school.
- Indoor activities: using an exercise video, dancing, playing games with soft sports balls, and having a game of "Hide and Seek".
- Outdoor activities: going to the playground, rollerblading, riding bikes, and playing hopscotch.
- Special occasion activities: playing crazy golf, visiting a water park or theme park, and going for a ramble in the countryside.

Keep an activity log Make a record of your child's activity for a week. You and your child can work on this together, noting what he or she likes to do, as well as how often they're done and how much time is spent in each active pursuit. This will enable you to track how much exercise your child gets.

Make a fitness contract This is one way to get an inactive teenager moving (see page 167). Through a contract, parent and child can set goals and develop strategies for how to reach them, working on them together.

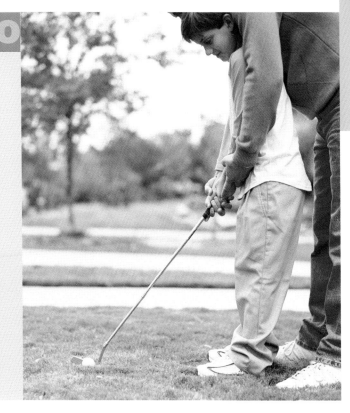

What's your child's fitness personality?

Personality traits and athletic ability combine to influence a child's attitude towards participation in sports and other physical activities. When children are very young, most tend to move around a lot and don't need to be reminded to exercise. But this may change as they get older.

Which of these three types best describes your child?

- The non-athlete: this child may lack athletic ability, lack interest in physical activity, or both.
- The casual athlete: this child, who is not a star player, is interested in being active, but is at risk of getting discouraged in a competitive athletic environment.
- The athlete: this child has athletic ability, is committed to a sport or activity, and likely to concentrate on practice time and intensity of competition.

The non-athletic child may need to limit sedentary activities, such as watching TV, using the computer, or playing video games. For the very athletic child, the difficulty may be finding more free time and rest time. If you understand the concepts of temperament and fitness type, you'll be better able to help your child find the right activities and get enough exercise – and find enjoyment in physical activity. For more discussion of this topic, see pages 143–145.

hard, like what they're doing, and get positive feedback from parents. Older children want to know they compare well to their peers, so getting a compliment from their coach in front of the entire team can make a big difference. Teenagers also get a boost from coach or teacher compliments, but as they near adulthood they begin to set their own goals and work to achieve them.

One way children can track their own success is to use a pedometer. This small device attaches at the waist and counts each step the child takes. The pedometer can be calibrated to properly measure the distance the child travels as well. (See page 63 to learn about goals you can set for your child, including a 10,000-step challenge, and ways to assess your child's fitness.)

Make sure it's fun

Can you create fun? It may sound odd, but researchers have come up with a list of factors that make physical activity fun for children. Some of them are:

- having positive interactions with peers and sports coaches, who offer praise and support;

- feeling proud of mastering a skill and feeling good because others have noticed;
- loving the way it feels to do the activity – to glide through the water while swimming or somersault through the air in gymnastics.

Finding that special "fun" activity can be the catalyst for a lifetime of physical fitness. Your child will simply want to keep doing it. Parents need to have fun too – for good reason: research has found that parents who themselves enjoy physical activity are more likely to encourage activity in their children. So don't just walk the walk – make sure you enjoy the walk too!

All kinds of activity

Including a variety of physical activities in a typical week – for example, walking to a friend's house, enjoying free play, and attending sports practices or classes – ensures that a child has an active and healthy lifestyle. To get your child to commit to this, you might try setting up an activity schedule and monitoring results with an activity log or, for teenagers, drawing up a fitness contract (see opposite).

Couch potatoes

In tracking activity, don't forget to note sedentary time, which can be the arch enemy of an active lifestyle. To encourage your child to increase his or her activity level, you may have to limit your child's "screen time" – the amount of time he or she spends watching TV, using the computer, or playing computer and video games. The average school-age child watches 11.4 hours of TV, videos, and DVDs a week and spends as much as four and a half more hours playing computer games. Add to that the time children spend reading or studying, and it totals up to a lot of inactivity.

Here are some useful guidelines:

● Children under two shouldn't watch any TV. Even the most educational programme isn't as beneficial as exploring and interacting with the world around them.

● Children older than two should be limited to one to two hours of "screen time" (either computer or TV) per day.

Of course, quality counts as well as quantity, so parents need to be aware of their children's favourite TV programmes and computer games. Monitor what your child watches on TV, including DVDs and videos. Also be informed about which computer software your child is using and which Internet sites are most often visited.

How to gauge fitness

Fitness is hard to measure, but the best way to start is by paying attention to how active your child is on a typical day. From toddlers to teenagers, children should be active every day, getting a mixture of structured activity and free play time. (See page 54 for recommendations.)

If you are keeping an activity log (see page 60), you have an easy way of checking to see if your child is getting enough exercise. The total can include any kind of activity, from cutting the grass or doing another household task to running around a track. If your child is getting less than the recommended amount, think of ways you can encourage him or her to boost active time.

Another way to help you to gauge your child's physical fitness is to use assessment tests that have been developed in the United States (see opposite). These tests measure a child's performance against that of the average for their age. Note, though, that children don't get fit simply by doing the assessment tests. They are able to succeed at the tests by being physically active in ways that enhance the three elements of fitness: endurance, strength, and flexibility. (For some exercises that will help improve your child's fitness, see pages 57–59.)

tips

Get them away from the TV

If you're finding it difficult to get your children away from the television, here are some ways to gradually decrease the time they spend watching it.

● Provide the weekly TV listings for your children and encourage them to choose the programmes they want to watch.

● Switch on the TV when the programme starts and turn it off when it's over.

● Provide alternatives, such as playing games or arts and crafts projects.

● Keep a supply of skipping ropes, balls, and other equipment to hand so that kids have easy access to them whenever they feel like playing.

● And no matter how much they beg for one, do not put a TV in your child's bedroom.

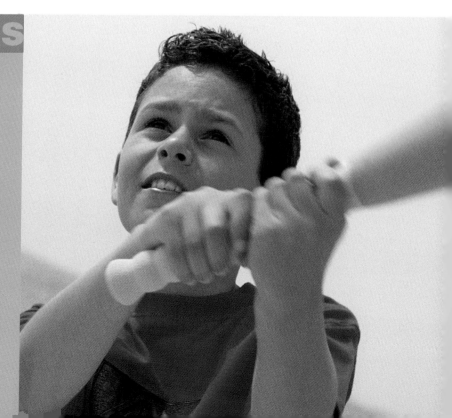

Assessing a child's **fitness**

In the United States, many schools and sports centres use a set series of targets to assess a school-age child's level of fitness. These targets are presented as challenges for children, and participation in the programme is the main goal. Children can use their baseline performance for comparison as they try to improve their skills.

The challenges use five tests of endurance, strength, and flexibility (see below) and measure the results achieved against the average performance for age. Children receive awards for achieving at the average level for their age and also just for participating in the challenge.

You might want to try using these tests to assess your child's fitness level. If the results show that your child isn't very fit, your response should be a gentle one. Congratulate your child for his or her efforts and offer encouragement and guidance about how to make improvements. The exercises on pages 57–59 are a good place to start. Just being more active every day – for example, taking more walks or more bike rides and climbing more at the playground – will also help your child improve fitness levels.

In addition, you could set a more specific goal for your child: that he or she must be active for at least 60 minutes a day, or walk 10,000 steps a day, at least five days a week for six weeks. Any physical activity done during the day, such as swimming or walking to a friend's house, can be included in the total. If your child is interested in trying this "10,000-step challenge", he or she could measure progress by using a pedometer (see page 61).

THE ASSESSMENT TESTS

- **Curl-ups (sit-ups)** Tests abdominal strength. The child lies on the floor, on back with legs bent and feet placed flat, arms crossed on chest. The child lifts chest towards knees until shoulders come off the floor, then lies back down. (See the photograph on page 59.)
- **Press-ups** Tests upper body strength. The child lies on the floor, face down, hands under shoulders, fingers straight, and knees bent (or legs straight and slightly apart). The child lifts body, keeping knees or toes on floor, until arms are straight, then lowers body to make a 90° angle at the elbows. (See the photograph on page 59.)
- **Sit and reach** Gauges lower back and leg flexibility. The child sits on the floor with legs straight and feet flat against a box. Reaching towards box while keeping legs straight, the test measures how far the child can bend forward.
- **1-mile run or walk** Tests heart and lung endurance. Younger children may be given shorter distances to complete in less time. Any child may choose to walk during part or all of the test, but no additional time is given.
- **Shuttle run** Gauges leg strength and agility. The child is timed while shuttling between two lines that are 9m (30ft) apart, retrieving and setting down blocks.

THE FITNESS TARGETS

AVERAGE AGE OF CHILD	CURL-UPS (SIT-UPS) (repetitions in 1 min)	PRESS-UPS (repetitions)	SIT AND REACH (distance)	1-MILE RUN/WALK (time)	SHUTTLE RUN (time)
BOYS					
Age 7	28	8	25cm (10in)	11:40 mins	12.8 secs
Age 10	35	14	25cm (10in)	9:48 mins	11.5 secs
Age 14	45	24	28cm (11in)	7:44 mins	9.9 secs
Age 17	44	37	34cm (13½in)	7:04 mins	9.4 secs
GIRLS					
Age 7	25	8	27cm (10½in)	12:56 mins	13.2 secs
Age 10	30	13	28cm (11in)	11:22 mins	12.1 secs
Age 14	37	10	33cm (13in)	10:06 mins	11.2 secs
Age 17	34	16	35cm (14in)	10:22 mins	11 secs

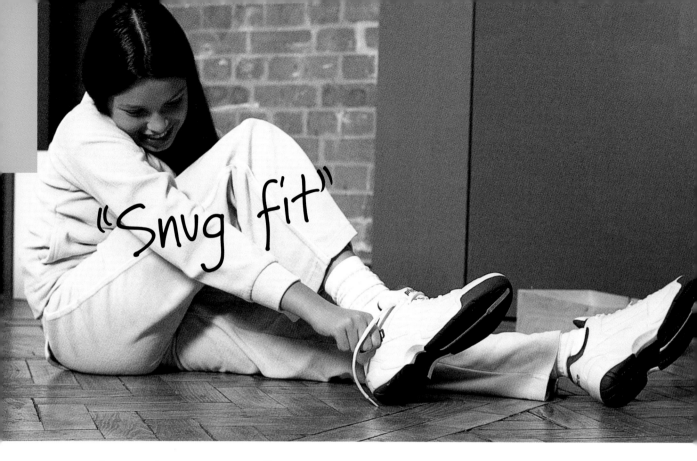

"Snug fit"

Playing safe

No matter how a child chooses to be active – or how old the child is – a parent needs to take the lead when it comes to sensible safety precautions and preventing injuries.

A sensible exercise programme

The principles of physical training are the same whether your child has ambitions to run a faster kilometre or just wants to start a gentle routine of daily walking. An exercise programme should include these four elements:

- a regular schedule of physical activity that's consistent from week to week;
- the right level of intensity so the child's body is working harder than it does when at rest, but without overdoing it, particularly if the child is normally inactive;
- a variety of activities so the child gets a good mixture of exercises and physical activities that improve endurance, strength, and flexibility;
- a gradual increase in the number of repetitions or in the amount of time spent exercising. Your child should make slow and steady progress towards a goal. Trying to go too fast can lead to injuries.

Good practice

Teach your child to exercise properly, from warm up to cool down. Before starting to exercise have your child warm up with five to ten minutes of brisk walking or slow jogging. Start slowly and gradually increase the pace. Warm-up exercises can help reduce muscle strain and prevent injuries. After exercise, cool down by stretching, which relaxes muscle groups and increases flexibility.

Take this same measured approach to help improve your child's fitness level. A very sedentary child might start slowly, with just one ten-minute walk a day. Add extra minutes each day or week, perhaps offering a pedometer as an extra incentive. You can also keep an activity chart for your child, and use it to set a baseline and choose a reasonable goal.

Some appealing activities are considered too dangerous for younger children because they lack the skills and judgement to do them safely. Here are some sensible recommendations to follow:

- Skateboards shouldn't be used by children under ten.
- Scooters shouldn't be used by children under eight.
- Trampolines should never be used at home.

The right gear

Protective equipment helps reduce the risk of injury by absorbing some of the blows that the body would otherwise take. An advantage of organized sports and club play is that most require appropriate protective clothing and adult supervision. At home, parents should provide the right protective equipment for their children's activities (see the list of suggested types of protective gear, below). Parents also need to be vigilant to ensure that children always wear the protective gear when playing or exercising and know how to use it properly.

This may be easier to require of younger children, but don't give up on the older ones. Playing hockey without pads or helmets is just asking for a trip to the accident and emergency department. And remember that gumshields not only protect the teeth but also help absorb the impact of hits to the mouth and jaw.

Older children may cast aside cycle helmets, believing they aren't cool or will mess up their hair. Parents must enforce the helmet rule regardless – and wear cycle helmets themselves. (For information about choosing a cycle helmet, to be sure that it fits well, see page 66.)

The sports gear **your child should be using**

Helmets protect the head when cycling, rollerblading, skateboarding, and playing various team sports. They are also recommended when children are skiing and snowboarding. Pads and guards protect specific parts of the body that are vulnerable to knocks and blows in sports such as basketball, football, hockey, and rugby. The protective equipment described below will minimize the risk of your child being injured while playing sport.

SPORT	EQUIPMENT
Basketball or netball	gumshield
Cricket	if male, a protective box. While batting: a helmet with face guard and eye protection; padded shorts; leg and thigh pads; arm guards
Football	shin guards or pads. For the goalkeeper: gloves
Hockey	mouth guard or gumshield; shin pads; gloves. For the goalkeeper: helmet with face guard and eye protection; padded body suit
Lacrosse	mouth guard. For the goalie: upper body protection; arm and leg pads. For older boys who play contact lacrosse, then helmet with attached mouth guard; gloves
Rollerblading	helmet; knee, wrist, and elbow pads
Rugby	gumshield; shoulder pads or upper body protection; scrum cap
Skateboarding	helmet; knee, wrist, and elbow pads

Take good care

Parents should supervise young children whenever they are outdoors and be extra careful when children are playing in the front garden or on the drive. Young children should be taught to ask for an adult's help to retrieve balls and to stay under control when riding bikes and trikes on the pavement so they don't drift into the road. Hassle your local councillor for traffic calming measures, such as a 20mph speed limit in your area, speed bumps or speed cameras, or creating a home zone. Use extra caution if children are playing outside at dusk, when it's difficult for drivers to see them.

Fun as it may be, it's best to discourage older children from rollerblading, skateboarding, and playing football or any other game in the street. Instead, provide them with transportation to a nearby park, playground, or playing field where they can have plenty of space.

While you're discouraging your child from playing in or near streets, you'll want to offer alternatives. Footpaths, cycle paths, and exercise tracks provide a safe environment for kids to walk or cycle without worrying about traffic.

Water safety

Children of all ages love the water, but water play and swimming can be dangerous: one of the major causes of accidental deaths in children younger than 14 is drowning.

Children between the ages of one and four are most at risk of drowning. Close and constant supervision is essential – drownings can occur in paddling pools and garden ponds, and can involve children who were out of their parents' sight for less than five minutes.

Swimming lessons are a good idea, though they are not a substitute for adult supervision.

- A child older than four is usually ready to learn how to swim. It's wise to use flotation devices – not water wings – to keep young children afloat in the water before they are able to swim on their own.
- Older children should be taught never to swim alone and that they should swim near lifeguards at pools.
- If someone other than a lifeguard is monitoring children, that person must know how to swim. This might sound obvious, but you'll want to be sure that babysitters, neighbours, and grandparents are capable of rescuing a child, if necessary.

Swimming goes hand in hand with bright, sunny days, so you'll want to take sun-safety precautions as well. Insist that children wear sun cream with a high sun protection factor (SPF) of 30 or above, and reapply it after swimming even if it's waterproof. Also encourage kids – especially those who are prone to sunburn – to wear hats that shield their heads and neck, and sunglasses to shield their eyes.

tips

The perfect fit

Cycle helmets, which are made from expanded foam polystyrene covered with moulded hard plastic, must fit well to protect the head in a fall. When choosing a helmet for your child:

- Pick one that fits snugly but comfortably on your child's head. The helmet should rest level on your child's head, not tilted forwards or backwards. Remove any hats or caps before putting the helmet on.
- Look for strong, wide straps that fasten snugly under the chin – no more than a finger's width should be able to fit beneath the strap when it is fastened correctly. Straps should be tight enough so that sudden pulling or twisting does not cause the helmet to move around on the child's head.
- If your child takes a significant fall, replace the helmet because it may have lost its effectiveness after taking a hit. Even if the helmet looks fine, it may be cracked inside, so throw it away and buy a new one.

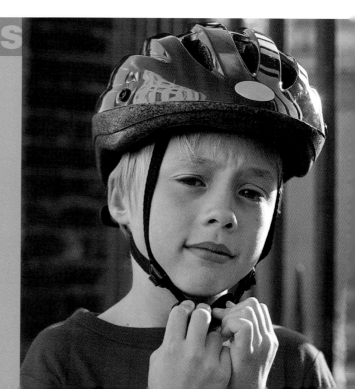

Drink for sport

It's important to be sure your child drinks enough before, during, and after exercise. A child needs water, or other fluids such as juice mixed with water, to prevent dehydration as well as heat-related illnesses like heat stroke and heat exhaustion.

Provide lots of liquid

Parents can help prevent injury in children of all ages by being on the lookout for dehydration. A child who is becoming dehydrated cannot perform at his or her best and is at greater risk of injury because energy, strength, and coordination may diminish.

Thirst is the first sign of dehydration, so offer your child some water to drink. But even if children satisfy their thirst, it may not be enough to replace all the fluid lost on a hot day. Other signs of dehydration include feeling lightheaded, rapid heartbeat, and dry mouth and lips.

Decreased frequency of urination is another sign of dehydration, as is urine colour. If your child is adequately hydrated, the urine should be a pale yellow colour. If your child's urine is dark or strong smelling, it could be a sign of dehydration. But this isn't the most practical way to monitor your child during sports practice on a hot day, so frequent water breaks are important.

Heat-related illness

Children may be at greater risk than adults for heat-related illnesses such as heat exhaustion (fatigue, weakness, and discomfort when overheated) and heat stroke (when the body becomes dangerously overheated). This is because children's bodies are less efficient at cooling down.

Look for these early signs of heat illness, which, if untreated, can progress to shock and loss of consciousness:

- pale skin
- headache
- rapid heartbeat
- nausea or vomiting
- muscle cramps
- goosebumps or excessive sweating
- fatigue, weakness, or dizziness.

Quenching thirst
Children of all ages need to drink plenty of fluids when playing or exercising – even more when the weather is hot. Water is the best choice to keep them hydrated.

To prevent heat-related illness, schedule breaks during exercise sessions and encourage your child to drink plenty of fluids; when the weather is warm limit activity during the hottest time of the day (usually 10 am to 2 pm); and be sure your child wears lightweight, loose-fitting clothing.

Anyone who cares for your child also should take steps to avoid putting the child at risk. This could include relatives, childcare workers, and sports coaches. In addition, be sure to teach your child to tell an adult if he or she starts to feel overheated and ill when playing or exercising. It's fine to work up a little sweat, but it's not okay to "play through" overexertion that could lead to illness.

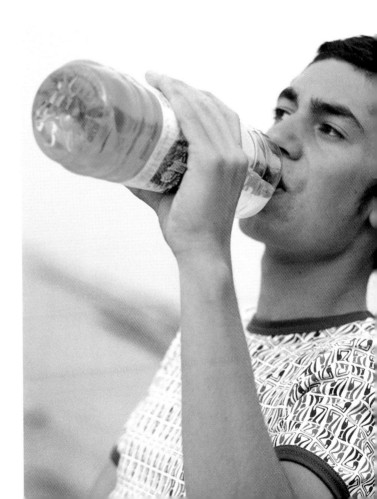

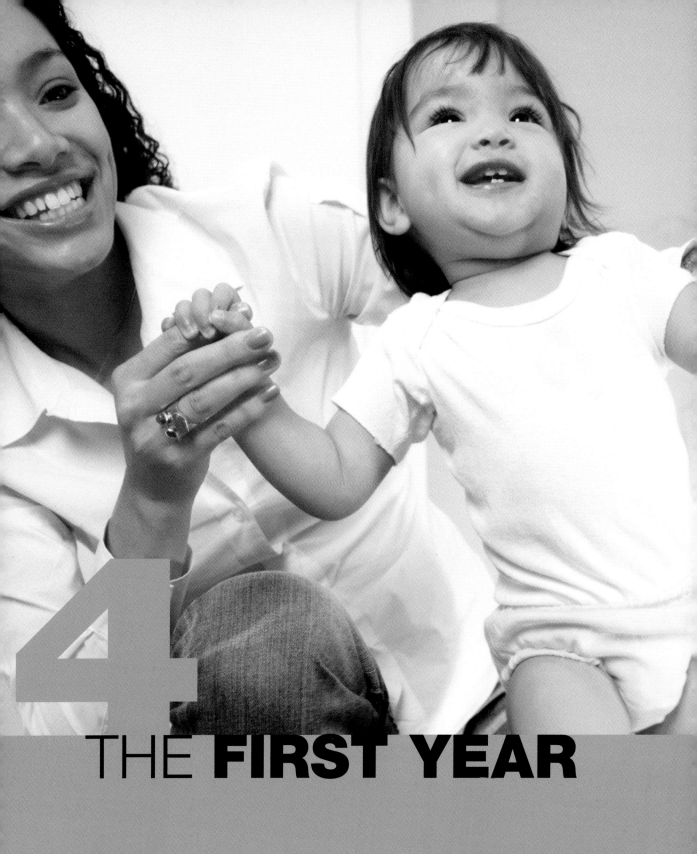

4 THE FIRST YEAR

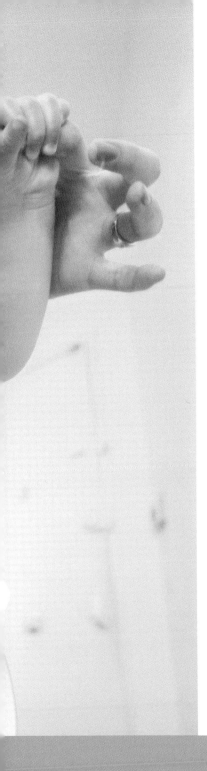

It all starts here. In these twelve months you can start **building a foundation of good health** for your baby. Learn how to provide **proper nutrition and the right activities** during this important first year.

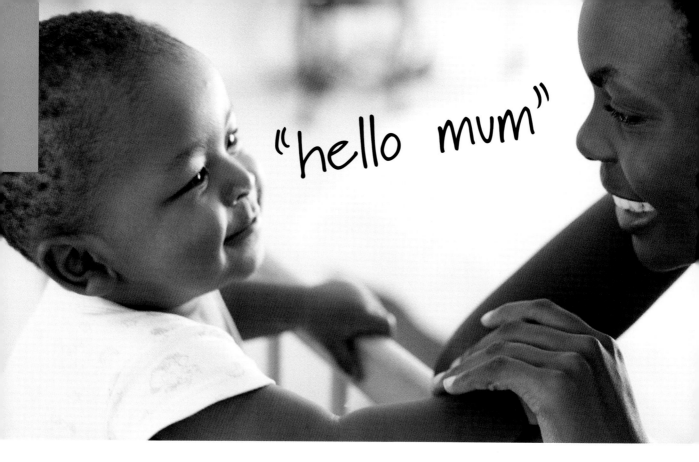

"hello mum"

Making a good start

Your baby begins life completely dependent on you, but in just 12 months' time that swaddled infant becomes a separate little person able to feed himself or herself and maybe even walk.

Do what comes naturally

Progress can be seen almost weekly as babies learn to lift their heads, roll over, sit up, crawl, cruise, and stand alone. Healthy eating and activity help a baby develop at this phenomenal rate, so parents often want to know exactly what to do and when to do it:

- How do I know my baby is eating enough?
- When do I introduce solid food?
- How can I encourage my child to crawl?

Though there are guidelines about feeding and activity that parents should know, much of what a baby needs parents do naturally as they love their child and begin a relationship with this fascinating new member of the family. A parent learns to respond to a child's needs, whether the baby is in need of a cuddle, hungry, or the nappy needs changing. This responsiveness helps the child feel secure.

Feeding your baby

When a baby cries, a parent's first thought may be to offer food. The trouble is, babies can't say whether they're hungry or not. But during a feed, a baby might turn his or her head away – a sign that he or she may have eaten enough. "Enough" changes dramatically during the first 12 months of life. Newborns start out needing only 500 calories per day, but that requirement grows to about 1000 calories by the end of the first year.

With time, parents can learn to spot cues that their baby is satisfied and even to distinguish a hungry cry from a tired one. By picking up your baby's cues – and responding in a sensitive way – you can help your child begin a healthy relationship with food. You may be concerned that you are underfeeding or overfeeding your baby. But, in fact, most babies take just what they need. Let your child use his or her innate ability to regulate food intake.

You can confirm that your baby is getting the right amount by watching his or her growth. At regular visits, your GP will monitor weight and length to see that the baby is growing as expected. Following an initial weight loss that occurs in the first week of life, healthy babies quickly regain this weight and thereafter gain about 200g (7oz) a week until three months of age, doubling their birth weight by about five months and then tripling it by the end of the first year.

Physical achievements to celebrate

Year one is a wondrous time as babies become more active. Your child grows from a curled-up infant into a baby who can sit unassisted, pull up to a stand, "cruise", and then walk.

To make tracks as they do, babies need stimulation and the opportunity to be active, but they don't "exercise". Watch for cues that your baby is ready to try new skills, so you can offer encouragement.

- If your five-month-old now can hold his or her head up and grasp objects, put a toy just out of reach, to challenge the baby.
- When you find your nine-month-old standing up in the cot, the child is showing you he or she is ready to take the next step. In a childproofed room, let the child stand holding on to the sofa to practise standing and cruising along the furniture.

For older children, it's important that parents are positive role models when it comes to physical activity. You may think this doesn't matter for your baby, and that he or she won't know whether you're snoozing on the sofa or out for a walk, with the baby in a pushchair, introducing him or her to the birds, squirrels, and big blue sky. At first your baby may seem oblivious to it all, but before long he or she will adjust to the pattern of the family routine. If that routine is an active one, everyone – parents and baby alike – will benefit.

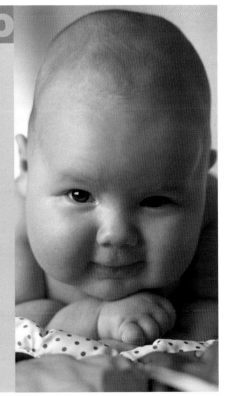

info

The overweight baby

Everyone loves a chubby baby, but if your doctor has told you your child is gaining too much weight, there's good reason to pay attention. Overweight babies are more likely to become overweight later in life, so consider whether a pattern of inactivity and overeating may have already begun. If you think this may be the case, never skip feeds or restrict your baby's feeds on your own. Seek advice from your child's doctor or health visitor instead.

Feeding too much?
Start by considering whether you could be overfeeding your baby. It can happen even to the best of parents, often because they are simply worried the baby is hungry or isn't eating enough. The trick is knowing when to stop. Be alert to cues that your baby is full, such

as slowing down and sucking with less enthusiasm, stopping, or turning away from the breast or bottle. If your baby is eating solid food, spitting it out may indicate he or she has had enough. (For feeding guidelines, see the chart on page 73.) And consider whether your baby may be getting excess calories from juices or puddings.

Not active enough?
An overweight baby might be getting too little activity. Be aware of how much time your child is spending in the cot, high chair, playpen, bouncer, car seat, or any other place that restricts movement. Even young babies need to move around and explore. When babies are overweight, it can make it more difficult for them to reach milestones, such as sitting up and pulling up to a stand.

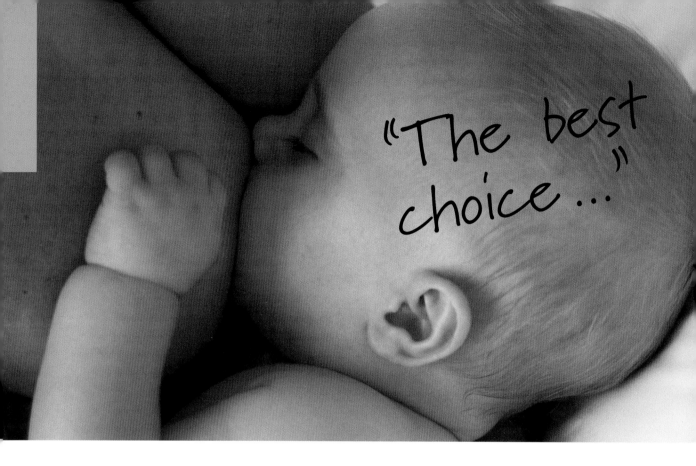

"The best choice ..."

Nutrition in the first year of life

From birth, parents and babies bond during feeding, which may have been first attempted minutes after delivery or not long after. It's about nutrition, but it's also a source of comfort and contentment.

What foods when?

The first decision parents need to make regarding nutrition is whether to breastfeed or bottlefeed. Breast milk is the ideal choice. If the mother can't breastfeed or chooses not to, babies who are bottlefed can grow up healthy too.

You'll begin introducing solid foods around six months and may start family food soon thereafter (see the feeding chart opposite). But even when your baby starts solid foods, breast milk or formula remain the most important source of nutrition throughout the first year.

The method of feeding changes dramatically during the first year. Babies learn to accept cereal and other food from a spoon and then endeavour to feed themselves, raking a

hand across the tray to scoop up some grub. And they'll play with food, getting it all over themselves in the process – as well as the floor, wall, and anywhere else in close enough proximity to the high chair.

But before you know it, your baby's accuracy will improve and he or she will become skilled enough to pick up a piece of dry cereal between forefinger and thumb, and pop it in their mouth. At this point babies are also deft enough to pick up things they shouldn't eat, so watch out!

By the time the family gathers to sing "Happy Birthday" to your one-year-old, he or she will be drinking from a feeder cup – though probably not without a few spills – and gamely eating a piece of that very first birthday cake.

sample **feeding schedule**

Use this chart as a guide – some babies may eat more or less. Check with your health visitor if you are unsure. A baby's first food should be rice-based cereal. Well-cooked eggs can be introduced after the age of six months.

AGE IN MONTHS	BREAST MILK	FORMULA	INFANT CEREAL (mixed with liquid)	VEGETABLES	FRUITS	MEAT, FISH, POULTRY, PULSES	POTATOES, PASTA, RICE
1	on demand	minimum 600ml (20floz)	none	none	none	none	none
2	on demand	minimum 600ml (20floz)	none	none	none	none	none
3	on demand	minimum 600ml (20floz)	none	none	none	none	none
4	on demand	minimum 600ml (20floz)	none	none	none	none	none
5	on demand	minimum 600ml (20floz)	none	none	none	none	none
6	on demand	minimum 600ml (20floz)	1–2 tbsp twice a day (rice cereal to start)	small amounts: about 1–2 tbsp, puréed	small amounts: about 1–2 tbsp, puréed	none	none
7	on demand	500–600ml (18–20floz)	2–3 tbsp twice a day	2–4 tbsp, puréed	2–4 tbsp, puréed	1–2 tbsp, puréed	1 tbsp, mashed
8	on demand	500–600ml (18–20floz)	2–3 tbsp twice a day	6–8 tbsp, puréed	2–4 tbsp, puréed	1–2 tbsp, puréed	1–2 tbsp, mashed
9	on demand	500–600ml (18–20floz)	3–4 tbsp twice a day	2–3 tbsp, puréed or mashed	3–4 tbsp, puréed or mashed	1–2 tbsp, puréed	2–3 tbsp, mashed
10	on demand	500–600ml (18–20floz)	3–4 tbsp twice a day	3–4 tbsp, mashed or finely chopped	3–4 tbsp, puréed, mashed, or finely chopped	2–4 tbsp, minced	4–5 tbsp, mashed or chopped
11	on demand	500–600ml (18–20floz)	4 tbsp twice a day	3–4 tbsp, mashed or finely chopped	3–4 tbsp, puréed, mashed, or finely chopped (fresh or cooked)	2–4 tbsp, minced or finely chopped	4–5 tbsp, mashed or chopped
12	on demand	500–600ml (18–20floz)	4 tbsp twice a day	3–4 tbsp, finely chopped	3–4 tbsp finely chopped (fresh or cooked)	3–4 tbsp, minced or chopped	5–6 tbsp, mashed or chopped

Feeding your baby in the early months

The menu is short for a newborn baby: breast milk or formula are the only choices because during these first six months babies usually don't need and shouldn't have anything else – no water, no juice, no regular milk, and no solid food.

Breastfeeding

Through breast milk a baby gets necessary vitamins and minerals and the amounts of other nutrients that nature intended. Breast milk also benefits a baby's immune system and may help reduce the risk of obesity later in life. While breastfeeding is the best nutritional choice for your baby, some supplements may be necessary, including vitamin D, fluoride, and iron. Check with your GP or health visitor.

Breastfed babies should eat when they're hungry, which may be often because breast milk is so easily digested. Early on a baby might want to feed every hour for periods, but in general feeds will be two to three hours apart. Even if a baby is feeding often, a parent may wonder if the child is getting enough. The number of wet and soiled nappies is a helpful indicator. Expect five or more wet nappies and two to five soiled ones every day during the first few weeks of life.

Overcoming any difficulties

While breastfeeding can be relaxing and become second nature over time, the early weeks can be difficult. Mothers may encounter problems, including breast soreness and inadequate milk production, or the baby may have trouble latching on to the breast. To ease sore nipples, squeeze out a few drops of milk and spread it on the nipple as a protective coating or try a nipple cream. Breast pain can be a sign of infection, so contact your doctor or health visitor if you are concerned.

Sucking is the best way to rev up milk production, so frequent feeds, or expressing milk between feeds, will help. Adjusting the way the baby latches on can help improve the milk supply and allow the baby to become a more efficient feeder. It can also make breastfeeding more comfortable. Be sure your baby takes the whole nipple into his or her mouth and begins sucking rhythmically.

Contact your doctor if your baby is not latching on successfully or not wetting nappies, or you have other concerns. Instead of just giving up and switching to bottlefeeding, get some professional guidance first.

Establishing closeness
For babies, breast milk is simply the perfect food, strategically packaged to require a lot of close, warm, snuggling time with mum.

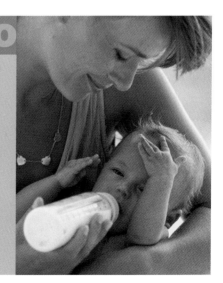

Comparing the benefits of breastfeeding and bottlefeeding

Breastfeeding
- requires no preparation or refrigeration
- costs little
- provides milk that is easily digested
- decreases baby's risk of allergy and protects against infection and other illnesses (antibodies)
- may reduce the risk of weight problems in future
- promotes bonding between mother and baby

Bottlefeeding
- offers more freedom and flexibility for the mother
- makes it easier to know how much the baby is getting
- may require fewer feeds because formula is digested more slowly than breast milk
- may make it easier to feed the baby in public places
- lets dad and other family members help feed the baby

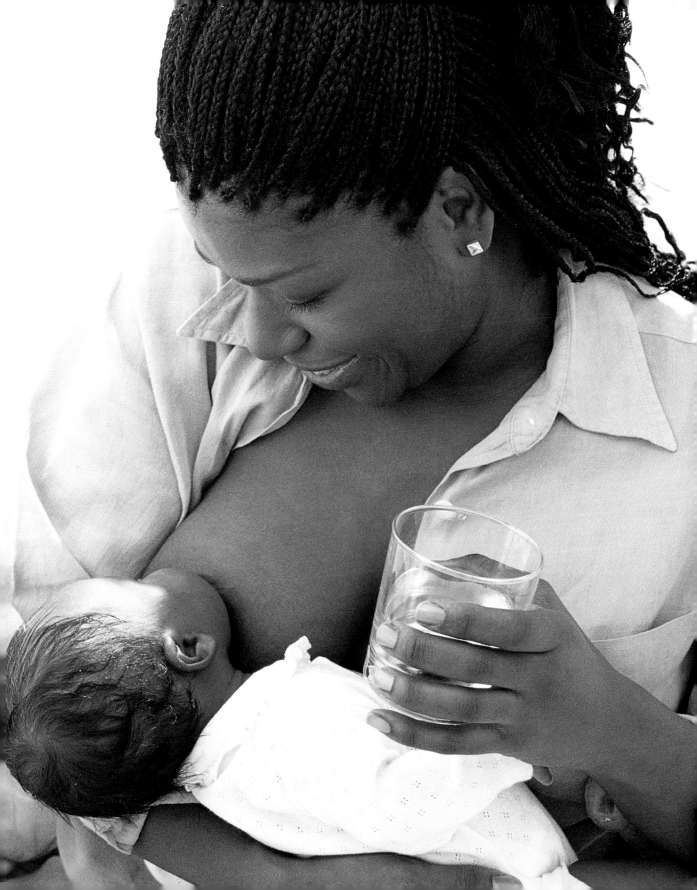

If possible, babies should be breastfed as long as possible, ideally until they are at least one year old. If you decide to change to bottlefeeding before then, it's important to choose the correct type of milk for your baby's age. There are many types of milk available, but up to six months of age the only milks suitable are breast milk and baby milk. Other types of milk are not suitable (unless recommended by a doctor) as they will not meet a baby's nutritional needs. From the age of six months you can use a follow-on milk.

The needs of breastfeeding mums

In the midst of all the attention being showered on the new baby, breastfeeding mothers also need to remember to take care of themselves.

- To meet her own nutritional needs as well as her baby's, a mum generally needs an additional 450–550 calories every day, for a total of 2200–2700 (depending on the mother's activity level and pre-pregnancy needs).
- A breastfeeding mum is the baby's source of vitamins and minerals, so it's crucial that she eat plenty of fruits and vegetables, as well as calcium-rich foods (to get an extra 550mg for a total of about 1250mg of calcium a day). She also should continue to take a prenatal vitamin that includes iron.
- While breastfeeding, a mum needs to drink lots of water and other fluids – especially before and after a feed.

Bottlefeeding

If you've chosen to bottlefeed your baby, you can be confident about meeting your infant's nutritional needs. Improvements in formulas have made them very close in nutritional value to breast milk. The two major types of infant formula are cow's-milk-based and soya-based. Your doctor will probably recommend which one to give your infant.

Most babies will do well on a cow's-milk-based formula, but talk with your doctor or health visitor if your child develops rashes or digestive problems that you think could be related to the formula. A lactose-free or soya-based formula may be recommended if lactose intolerance is suspected. There are also hypoallergenic formulas available for babies who are allergic to cow's milk. Be sure to consult your doctor or health visitor before switching formulas.

Formula based on cow's milk does, of course, contain cow's milk, but it has been modified to be more easily digested and nutrionally complete. Babies should not be given the cow's milk you buy in the supermarket until they are at least one year old because it lacks the vitamins and nutrients babies need to grow. It also has too much protein for babies to digest and too little of the fat a baby needs for normal growth and development.

Formulas are designed to meet a baby's nutritional needs and should not be diluted with anything else, or replaced by any other liquid, unless the doctor has told you to do so.

tips

Winding a baby

Babies often swallow air while feeding, especially the very hungry ones who were crying beforehand. Because of this it's a good idea to stop during a feed to wind your child, even before he or she starts fussing. A fussing baby will end up swallowing more air, which may make the child feel even more uncomfortable. Winding your baby regularly should also reduce the amount of regurgitating.

Use gentle taps on the baby's back or slowly rock your upright baby's body forwards and back to encourage a burp. Another option is to lay your baby across your lap, face down, and gently pat his or her back. If your baby doesn't burp,

don't worry. Just go back to feeding if he or she is still hungry, and try again at the end of the feed.

- For breastfeeding mums, take some time to wind your baby when you switch breasts.
- If you are bottlefeeding, wind your baby once or twice during each feed, stopping to do so first after about half of the formula is taken, or as needed.

Don't be overzealous about winding your baby. It could backfire and lead to more regurgitating. Any air that is not burped out will pass through the baby's intestinal tract and come out the other end.

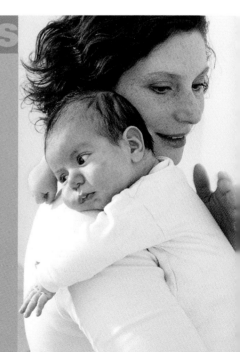

What kind of formula?

You can buy formula prepared and ready to use or as a powder or concentrate that needs to be mixed with water. They are similar in nutritional value, as long as they are prepared according to the manufacturer's directions. Improperly prepared formula can interfere with a baby's growth and may endanger health.

Once you have chosen a formula, you'll need a delivery system – a bottle and teat. You have a variety to choose from. It's important to wash, rinse, and sterilize the bottles and teats, as well as any equipment used to make up the feeds, to protect your baby from harmful germs. If you're unsure how to do this, ask your health visitor for advice.

Use freshly boiled and cooled tap water to make up feed. Water that has been repeatedly boiled or artificially softened is not suitable, nor is water that has been passed through some jug water filters. If you're unsure about the water supply – for example if you are travelling abroad – then you may choose to use boiled bottled water. The mineral composition of bottled waters varies, so ask your healthcare professional which ones are suitable for babies.

How much to feed and when

Though formula is digested more slowly than breast milk, bottlefed babies still feed often, usually every two to three hours in the early months. Like breastfed babies, they should be fed on demand. Newborns generally drink a little more than 60ml (2floz) of formula a day for each 450g (1lb) of body weight. A 3.6-kg (8-lb) baby will drink about 600ml (20floz) a day, feeding about six times a day. Babies who drink smaller amounts tend to feed more frequently. As they get older, babies will drink larger amounts and may feed less frequently.

Because it's less work to get the milk from a bottle, it's easier to overfeed a bottlefed baby. Be cautious of teats that flow too quickly, and take breaks during feeds so your baby has a chance to sense being full. You might try filling the bottle 30ml (1floz) beyond the normal feed so you are able to offer the extra if your baby wants more.

Make the most of feeding time. Find a comfortable spot and nestle your baby's head on the inside of your bent elbow. Never use a bottle prop – it carries the risk of choking and encourages your child to sleep with a bottle in the mouth. Avoid putting a child to sleep with a bottle, even when he or she can hold it unassisted. It can cause serious tooth decay.

Getting it right

Eating patterns will vary from baby to baby, so it's important to be flexible and responsive to your child. Growth spurts also occur, triggering periods of increased appetite. During these times a baby may go off his or her normal schedule to keep up with the demands of this growth. Even a very young baby will let you know whether he or she is hungry or has had enough. The trick is paying attention to the cues and not forcing a baby to eat beyond his or her hunger.

Babies who are getting enough seem satisfied after a feed. A baby might show he or she is full by slowing down the feeding, stopping, or turning away from the breast or bottle. Pay attention to how your baby tries to get this message across. Some babies continue to suck after they are full, but usually with less enthusiasm. This could lead to overfeeding, particularly for a baby who is bottlefed. Most babies are comforted by sucking, so a parent may want to encourage thumb-sucking or try a dummy. But don't use a dummy as a substitute for feeding a hungry baby.

The baby who regurgitates a lot

Regurgitating is an expected part of an infant's early eating. This usually becomes less frequent by six months and is nearly gone by nine or ten months. Regurgitating a small amount (less than 30ml/1floz) isn't cause for concern as long as it occurs within an hour of a feed and doesn't bother the baby, who is growing normally. Minimize regurgitating by:

- feeding the baby before he or she gets very hungry (a hungry baby is likely to swallow air and overfeed);
- keeping the baby in a semi-upright position (head raised) during the feed and for an hour after eating;
- winding the baby regularly;
- avoiding overfeeding;
- checking the flow of liquid from the bottle's teat to make sure the hole is not too large or too small; the liquid should drip slowly, not pour out of the hole;
- not jostling or playing vigorously with the baby right after a feed.

Sometimes regurgitating can be a sign of another problem. Talk with your GP or health visitor if your child is frequently irritable, regurgitating large amounts, or vomiting forcefully, as well as if your child seems to be losing weight or not gaining weight as expected. Also get medical attention without delay if your child has a fever or shows any signs of dehydration (such as not wetting nappies).

Introducing solid foods

"When are you going to give that baby some real food?" That's what well-meaning relatives and friends want to know. But young babies simply aren't ready to eat solid foods. And giving them solids too soon can increase the risk of food allergies.

The right time for solids

When you were a child, the doctor may have told your mother to give you cereal at two months – maybe even mixing it in with your bottle of formula. Today most experts recommend waiting until six months to offer cereal or any other solid food. Here's why: to eat solid food an infant needs good head and neck control and should be able to sit up. Your baby may not be able to do these things until four to six months. Before then babies will push food out of their mouths just as quickly as you put it in. This is a natural reflex that is lost by about six months, after which it becomes easier for them to start eating solid foods.

By taking it slowly with solid foods, you'll also reduce the risk of your baby developing food allergies, especially if allergies run in your family. (See opposite for more about

Feeding infant cereal
Use a spoon and offer small quantities so your baby can learn the mechanics of moving food to the back of the mouth and coordinating swallowing.

allergenic foods and when to introduce them.) A baby's developing immune system will be better able to handle new foods after the age of six months.

Infant cereal

Baby rice cereal is usually given first because it's less likely to cause an allergic reaction. Initially it is mixed with breast milk or formula so it's more of a liquid than a paste. Talk with your child's doctor or health visitor about the right age to begin solid foods and how to phase them in. (See page 73 for a feeding guide.)

Though your mother and grandmother may swear by it, never give infant cereal in a bottle unless a medical condition requires it. Babies who are fed this way may get too many calories and become overweight. Eating cereal from the bottle also can interfere with the transition to other solid foods. Introduce infant cereal by feeding your baby with a small spoon and be sure to take it slow. It's important never to force food into a baby's mouth.

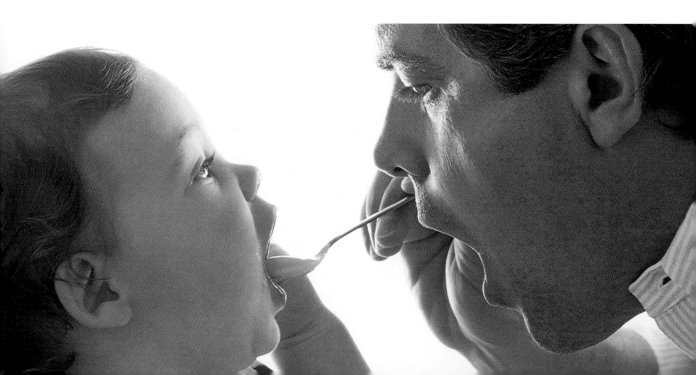

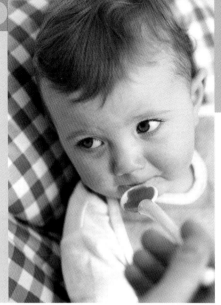

info

Allergenic foods

Some foods can cause allergic reactions and should not be introduced to young children. A child is at higher risk for food allergies if one or more of his or her close family members have allergies or allergy-related conditions, especially food allergies, eczema, or asthma. (For more information about food allergies, see page 174.) Waiting until the child is a little older to introduce these foods may help prevent lifelong allergies, so talk with your child's doctor about this.

Here are recommended ages for introducing allergenic foods to children at normal risk of developing an allergy and those at higher risk.

FOOD	NORMAL RISK	HIGHER RISK
Gluten (eg wheat and oats)	6 months	12 months
Citrus fruits	6 months	2 years
Fish and shellfish	6 months	3 years
Eggs	6–9 months	2 years
Nuts and peanut butter	2 years	3 years

Babies won't be very efficient eaters when they first start eating infant cereal. In fact, they may eat as little as a tablespoonful. It takes time for a baby to learn how to take food from a spoon and you may need to experiment with the cereal's consistency. Strive to keep the experience calm and pleasant by choosing a good time of day when the baby is alert, interested, and not overly hungry.

When starting infant cereal, you may notice a change in your child's stools. It's okay if the baby doesn't have a bowel movement every day as long as stools are soft. If the baby's stools are hard, dry, or difficult to pass, talk with your doctor or health visitor.

After your baby has tried rice cereal, you can then gradually introduce your baby to different tastes by adding vegetable and fruit purées to his or her diet (see page 80).

One new food at a time

When introducing new foods to your baby, it is important to give him or her one food at a time, and to wait several days before trying something else new. This can get confusing, so you may want to introduce one new food a week and select a day of the week as "new food day". If your baby doesn't seem to like a particular food, reintroduce it at subsequent meals. It may take quite a few tries before your child finally warms up to a particular food, so don't give up after the first or second attempt.

Introducing new foods one at a time also gives you an opportunity to see if your baby is allergic to it. If your baby is allergic, you may notice one of the following:
- a rash
- diarrhoea
- excess wind
- fussiness after eating.

For more severe allergic symptoms, such as hives or breathing difficulty, get medical attention straight away. (For more information about food allergies, see page 174.) Whether the reaction is mild or severe, don't try the offending food again until you talk with your GP or health visitor.

Some experts suggest that vegetables should be the first foods offered because they fear babies won't like vegetables if they've already enjoyed sweet fruits. But there's no evidence that giving vegetables first produces veg-loving kids, so parents are free to start with a fruit if they choose. That's not to say you should neglect vegetables. One approach is to alternate fruits and vegetables. If your baby tries bananas or pears one week, you might offer carrots or avocado the next week. In this way, you'll be working towards introducing a wide variety of fruits and vegetables.

These first forays into the eating world begin to establish food preferences – your child's likes and dislikes – for years to come. Using a patient, gentle approach, you can help your baby develop a taste for many nutritious foods.

When should my baby have juice?

Juice can be given after six months of age, but remember that it adds extra calories without the balanced nutrition found in formula and breast milk. Also, drinking too much juice may contribute to overweight or cause diarrhoea in infants. Later it can contribute to tooth decay. When you introduce juice, follow these recommendations:

- Offer juice in a feeder cup or regular cup, not in a bottle.
- Limit the quantity of juice to 120ml (4floz) per day.
- Start with juices of the fruits your child has already tried and tolerated.
- Serve only 100-percent fruit juice, not juice drinks or powdered drink mixes (which are sweetened).

Baby food

Parents can buy ready-prepared baby foods or make their own, using a food mill or food processor. Commercial baby food has some advantages, especially if you choose brands that avoid fillers and added sugar. Ready-prepared baby foods in jars also don't need refrigeration and are easy to take with you. Processing reduces the likelihood of exposure to pesticides, but if you are concerned consider organic alternatives, although they cost more. (For more information about organic foods, see page 47.) When preparing your own baby foods, be sure to follow the guidelines below.

Whichever type of baby food you choose, texture and consistency are important considerations. At first babies need to eat finely puréed single foods (for example, just apple purée, not apples and pears mixed together). Later,

after they've had a variety of foods, they can have two foods mixed together but still puréed. At nine to ten months, many babies are ready for coarser, chunkier textures, including more family foods, but the transition should be gradual. Just as babies develop other skills, they need time to work on the various skills related to eating: accepting a bite of food, controlling food in the mouth, using the jaws to chew, and coordinating their swallow.

Certain foods, such as mashed potatoes or puréed cooked carrots, are often the first family foods a baby is offered. But don't give heavily seasoned foods to a baby or dishes that contain foods the baby hasn't already tried. Also avoid those foods that are likely to cause allergic reactions (see the list of these on page 79).

What's my baby's temperament?

Even as a baby, a child has a unique personality that will become more fully developed over the months and years to come. An infant or child may be described as easy-going or difficult or, more often, somewhere in between. Your child's temperament – the inherent way he or she interacts with the world – will influence mealtime.

By understanding your infant's temperament, you can avoid conflict and help him or her adapt to changes, such as learning to eat solid food or trying new foods. For example, an infant who is sensitive to the texture of food may initially reject a new fruit. Don't give up. Offer the new fruit in small amounts or mix the new fruit with an accepted cereal. Alternatively, simply try introducing it on another day.

info

Home-made baby purées

If you want to make your own baby purées, be sure to follow these guidelines:

- Don't add salt or sugar to any food being prepared for babies.
- Steam or bake fruits or vegetables instead of boiling, which washes away nutrients.
- If you aren't going to use all of a baby purée right away, or you have prepared some purées in bulk, freeze them rather than bottling. For freezing, use sterilized ice cube trays at first and later small pots such as empty yogurt cartons.
- Adhere to food safety rules, such as frequent hand-washing, keeping utensils clean, and keeping hot foods hot and cold foods cold.

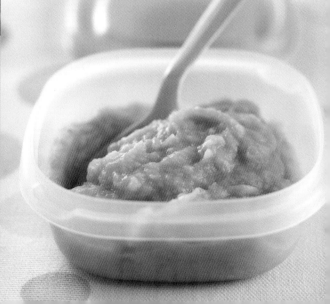

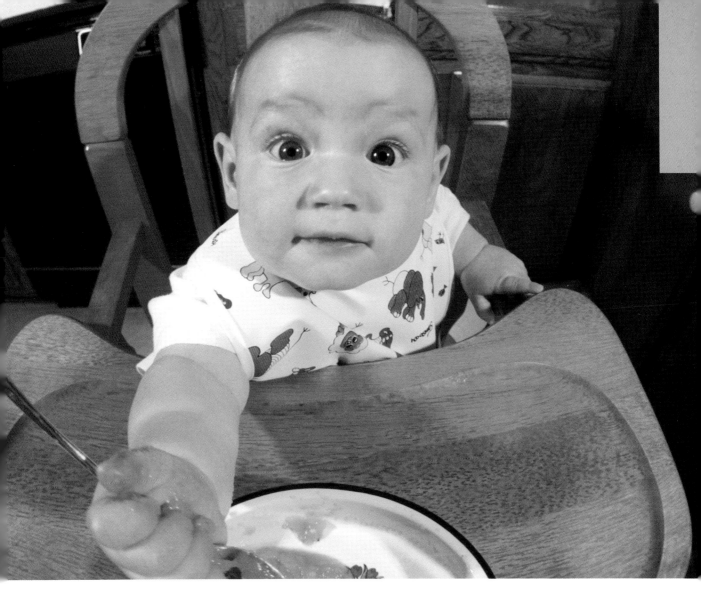

To learn more about your baby's temperament, ask yourself the following questions:

- Is my baby always on the go or laid back?
- Is my baby unpredictable or does he or she follow a regular schedule?
- How does my baby react to new situations?
- Is my baby easily distracted or able to focus?
- What's my baby's general mood?
- Is my baby hypersensitive to light, noise, touch, or textures?

A more sensitive child may not like your "playing airplane" with the spoon to get the food into his or her mouth. On the other hand, if your baby thrives on stimulation, feel free to have some fun as long as the focus remains on eating.

One of the gang
Pull the baby's high chair right up to the table at family mealtimes. You'll notice that he or she will be increasingly interested in what everyone else is having for dinner.

In addition to being spoon-fed, your baby may like to take charge a bit by feeding himself or herself a rusk and holding – though not really using – his or her own spoon while you do the actual feeding. Once your baby grows accustomed to eating, have him or her join the rest of the family at mealtimes. It may seem more efficient (and less messy) to feed the baby separately, but this is a missed opportunity. By the age of nine months or so, your baby will start to enjoy being part of the family action.

Feeding themselves at ten to twelve months

Your child's relationship with food is about to get messier and more delicious. He or she is now old enough to leave those baby purées behind in favour of foods with real texture – and to start eating them without help from mum and dad.

Discovering tastes and textures

Now that they're joining the rest of the family at the table, older babies are ready – and often willing – to try more family foods. This will mean additional work for whoever is preparing the meals for the family, but often dishes can be adapted for the baby. For instance, your baby can have some of the courgettes you're serving for dinner, as long as you cook his or her portion just a little longer – until it's soft – and cut it into small enough pieces for the baby to handle. Soups are another good choice. (See opposite for some ideas on how to cook a special soup for your baby.)

While your child's menu is getting more exciting, so is his or her means of eating. The older baby is able to use developing fine motor skills to pick up small pieces of food. During these months, your baby will be able to take hold of food between index finger and thumb in a pincer grasp. Sometimes the baby will eat the food, sometimes not. The pincer grasp will start out a little clumsy, but with practice it will soon evolve into a masterful and efficient skill.

Offer your infant a choice of "safe foods" (see below for suggested finger foods) and let your child feed himself or herself. Do this as much as possible. Though it can be a little slow, it's consistent with how you want to approach feeding throughout childhood: you present the child with healthy food and the child decides what to eat, or even whether to eat at all. It's normal to worry that your infant isn't getting enough, but remember how small his or her body and tummy are. Portions must be small.

The small portions should include food that has been cut up into small pieces. The size of the pieces varies depending on the food's texture. A piece of chicken, for instance, needs to be smaller than a piece of banana, which even a pair of baby gums will quickly smash.

Some children are more sensitive to texture and may reject anything coarse, such as meat. Parents may worry if their child doesn't seem to like meat, but this is not a concern with such a young child because the baby's protein needs are still being met through breast milk or formula.

tips

Which finger foods are safe for my baby?

At around ten months, babies can start trying finger foods. But which foods are best? If you are unsure about a food, pop it in your mouth and ask yourself these questions:

Does it melt in the mouth? Some dry cereals will melt in the mouth as will biscuits that are light and flaky.

Is it cooked enough so that it mushes easily? Well-cooked vegetables and fruit will mush easily as will canned fruit and vegetables (choose those that are canned without added sugar or salt).

Is it naturally soft? Cottage cheese, grated cheese, and small pieces of tofu are soft.

Can it be gummed? Pieces of ripe banana and well-cooked pasta can be gummed.

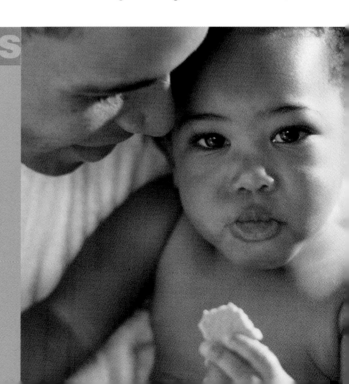

To introduce meats, start with well-cooked minced meats or very small pieces of cooked meats such as chicken. If your child doesn't like meat (or any other food), don't let that stop you from offering it again. Present it, but don't force your baby to eat it. This allows the baby the opportunity to grow more accustomed to the food and eventually accept it.

Hold the sweets

At first bite, your baby probably will love the taste of cake, ice cream, and other sweets, but do not introduce them now. Your child needs to eat nutrient-rich foods instead of consuming empty calories found in desserts and other sugary treats. It's tempting to want to see the baby's reactions to some of these foods, but now is not the time. Grandparents and others may want to rush your baby into trying chocolate gateau or some other family favourite. Politely and firmly explain that the baby isn't ready for those foods. If granny persists and says you had your first bite when you were an infant, blame this tough stance on your doctor. The doctor won't mind.

Take care with finger foods

Eating with the fingers is fun and rewarding for the older infant, but it's important to avoid foods that can cause choking. Parents and childminders also can help prevent choking by supervising the baby while he or she is eating. Foods that are choking hazards include:

- pieces of raw vegetable and hard fruits
- raisins, whole grapes, and cherry tomatoes (instead, serve grapes and cherry tomatoes cut into quarters)
- chipolatas (peel and cut these into very small pieces)
- breadsticks and toast
- pieces of hard cheese
- whole nuts

A middle-of-the-night feed

Just as you are enjoying your baby's new eating habits, you may be surprised that – out of the blue – he or she wants a bottle in the middle of the night. But something other than hunger may be the cause if your child has started awakening during the night again. Infants at this age are aware enough of their world to notice when parents are not around. They may express this realization quite loudly in the middle of the night and parents may assume that the crying means their baby is hungry.

Q: My ten-month-old isn't ready for most food I cook for my family. What's a good meal to serve her?

A: Sometimes you can adapt the family's meal to suit your baby's limited palate, but other times you'll need to cook something separate. Thick vegetable soup is easy to prepare and a batch can be divided into small containers and kept in the freezer.

Start by lightly cooking vegetables in a little olive oil. Include only those vegetables your child has already tried. Carrots, courgettes, potatoes, and sweet potatoes are good choices for soup as are canned peas or green beans. Cut all vegetables into very small pieces.

For protein, add small pieces of chicken, tofu, or kidney beans. And don't forget some pasta. Choose a pasta shape that will be easy for the baby to pick up, such as twists or small shells. Add enough formula milk to bring the soup to the right consistency for your baby and cook until everything is soft. Serve the soup in a shallow bowl so your child can pick up the pieces and enjoy them.

If your baby was previously fine without an overnight feed, he or she might just need some reassurance. It's normal for an infant at this age to experience separation anxiety. If your baby wakes up, go to him or her. Pat your baby on the back, calm him or her down, and perhaps offer a comfort item such as a special blanket. But take care not to turn it into playtime, and try your best to avoid offering a middle-of-the-night feed because it can disrupt everyone's sleep and also may lead to a pattern of overeating.

Drinking on their own

By 12 months, a baby is ready for the switch from formula to cow's milk. If you've made it to the one-year mark with breastfeeding, congratulate yourself. You can continue breastfeeding for as long as you like or you can stop now.

You probably have already introduced the feeder cup to your baby, so let him or her keep working at using it. Little by little, cut back on the use of the bottle. This might be a tough transition for your child so don't rush it. Offer praise when your child sips from a cup because it's an important step towards eating like a big kid.

Activity for babies

The first year of a child's life is filled with the most amazing physical achievements – a series of predictable milestones. Like building blocks, each new skill provides the foundations for the next one.

Encouraging physical activity

Guidelines have been developed to encourage physical activity in babies. And those guidelines are very easy to follow. Babies need no formal programmes, the experts say; they simply need the daily opportunity to explore their environment. These guidelines apply to all babies, wherever they are cared for – at home, at a relative's house, or by a childminder. What children should have are a safe environment, room to explore, and a chance to use their muscles.

A young infant needs opportunities to develop head and neck strength. Next babies work on the strength in their trunks, which allows them to sit up at around six months. And nearing the end of the first year, babies want to seize every opportunity to move, whether it's by scooting, crawling, creeping, cruising, or walking.

The guidelines caution against letting babies spend too much time in confined spaces, such as car seats, pushchairs cots, and bouncing chairs. These places and devices can discourage physical activity because babies are restrained from moving and exploring. Instead, let your baby spend time trying out newly acquired skills, from reaching for a rattle to sitting without support and then taking first steps.

New parents are often easy targets for advertisers selling the latest toy or gadget designed to educate and entertain their precious baby. But you can provide enriching experiences without spending much money. Expensive toys, baby massage classes, and videos that introduce classical music or art are not necessary for healthy physical and cognitive development.

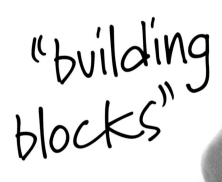

"building blocks"

Baby **development chart**

Your knowledge of normal infant development can help you encourage your child to be active and practise new skills, as well as having a lot of fun. Strengthening muscles and mastering these basic skills are the first steps towards lifelong physical activity. Your GP or health visitor can help you to understand your baby's development and which skills to look for next. There's no need to rush to the next stage. With support from their parents, babies will progress and develop successfully at their own pace.

AGE	WHAT BABIES CAN DO	RECOMMENDED ACTIVITIES
0–3 months	<ul><li>focus and follow objects, especially faces and brightly coloured or shiny toys</li><li>spontaneously wave arms and kick legs</li><li>raise head while on tummy</li><li>swipe for dangling objects</li><li>hold rattle placed in hand</li><li>smile and coo</li></ul>	while supervising, place baby on tummy to strengthen neck and shoulders; try an infant gym with dangling objects; put a rattle in the baby's hand
3–6 months	<ul><li>on tummy, prop self up and lift head</li><li>roll over</li><li>reach for and grasp objects</li><li>hold head steady while sitting</li><li>sit with support</li><li>laugh</li></ul>	continue tummy time; let baby sit supported on your lap; let baby reach for favourite toys and objects
6–9 months	<ul><li>sit without support</li><li>sit and pivot</li><li>stand with support</li><li>start to use finger and thumb to grasp objects</li><li>wave bye-bye</li><li>babble</li></ul>	keep a variety of toys within baby's reach in a safe play area; help baby pull up to stand; play Peek-a-Boo
9–12 months	<ul><li>get on hands and knees</li><li>crawl, scoot, or creep</li><li>pull up to stand</li><li>cruise along furniture</li><li>stand alone</li><li>first steps – maybe</li><li>say "mummy" and "daddy"</li></ul>	help pull up to stand; hold baby's hands and practise walking; let baby climb stairs with supervision; offer push-and-pull toys; sing action songs such as "Pat-a-Cake"

Babies want and need to spend time with the people who love them, who are the best teachers to help them with their developing skills. Looking at books together, singing songs, or going for a pushchair ride on a sunny day are wonderful experiences at a very reasonable price.

Being active is important, but don't forget that all babies need rest time too. After an energetic day of moving around, banging blocks together, playing Peek-a-Boo, and singing, take some time to turn down the lights and cuddle with your baby in your favourite rocking chair. The peaceful moments will be good for you both and will reinforce the baby's feelings of security and love.

Sensible safety precautions

Here are a few things to remember and steps to take before your baby becomes more mobile.

- Don't leave babies unattended on beds, sofas, or tables. Normally, infants start rolling over at four to six months, but even newborns can fall after unexpectedly kicking and turning, squirming, or rolling.
- Place stairgates at the top and bottom of all staircases. Stairs are often the reason why babies and toddlers get injured. Be sure to keep gates closed at all times.

- Use the safety strap on swings, pushchairs, and high chairs. Without a T-strap, which goes between a baby's legs, the child can get stuck or slip out and fall from these devices. Older children may stand up and fall over.
- Keep curtains, cords, and tablecloths out of a baby's reach. Between six and nine months, babies are eager to pull up to a stand and they will use anything they can get hold of to do it. They can be injured by falling objects or get tangled in cords.
- Don't use a baby walker. Walkers on wheels don't help babies learn to walk any sooner, and in fact they may delay walking because they don't encourage the baby to use the muscles involved in walking. On top of that, they're dangerous and are often the cause of serious falls down stairs. Choose a stationary walker or exercise saucer instead.
- Don't use borrowed baby safety equipment or buy used equipment from a car boot sale. These items aren't bargains because they are old and often don't have the instructions that inform parents how to use them correctly. Even products that are just a few years old may not reflect the latest in safety design and buyers won't know if the item has been recalled.

tips

Making childcare arrangements

Because children can spend many hours in childcare, it's important to know that your childminder understands the importance of being active – even for infants. When making a choice, look for a childminder who:

- understands physical development (such as when a baby is ready to roll over, sit with support, or pull up to a stand), so the childminder can help your child develop new skills;
- understands cognitive development, so the childminder knows which activities are right for your child's age and how to foster learning;
- limits the amount of time a baby spends in cots, high chairs, bouncing chairs, and other equipment that restricts movement;
- provides a safe environment so that your baby can explore freely;
- encourages lots of activity through interaction, singing, and playing;
- discourages the use of TV, videos, and DVDs as a means of keeping a baby entertained.

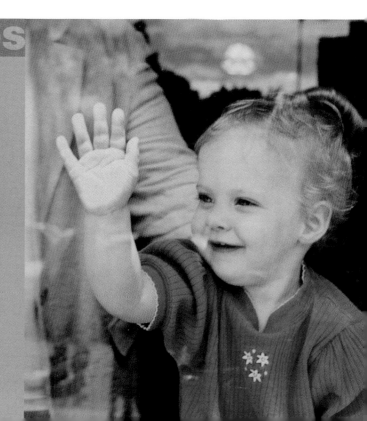

Kicking and smiling in the first three months

Though it may seem strange to think about "activity" for such a young baby, even at this early age babies do move their bodies. They wave and kick in a jerky way, but these movements increase their flexibility and strengthen muscles.

Signs of progress

New parents often talk about how they simply stare at their baby, wondering at this little person. During the first two months babies seem to do little more than sleep and eat, but here and there you'll begin to see glimpses of your child's unique self. Your child will start to recognize your face and smile at the sound of your voice.

As you care for your baby you are laying the foundation for a strong committed relationship, which is essential to your baby's development. Progress starts in small ways with this tiny infant, taking little steps towards important milestones that are reached during the first six months of life, such as holding his or her head steady, rolling over, grasping objects, and sitting up with support.

By two to three months, a baby is able to do more and is increasingly interested in the world. The child can swipe at objects, bring a hand to his or her mouth, and grasp a toy. Soon your baby may realize he or she is the one causing the rattle to make noise – quite a discovery!

Tummy time

While awake, it's important for your baby to spend some time on his or her tummy, to help strengthen the neck and shoulders. Some parents are concerned about doing this because they have been instructed to avoid placing their baby on his or her front to prevent Sudden Infant Death Syndrome (SIDS). It is true that babies should not be put down to sleep face down because of the increased risk of SIDS, but when the child is awake, alert, and supervised "tummy time" is safe and beneficial.

Babies need constant supervision while they are on their tummies, in case they tire out and need a parent to pick them up or flip them over. Start by trying tummy time a few times a day, but keep these sessions brief because your

baby may get frustrated in this position. As the baby gets better at this skill, he or she will enjoy it more and just might show off another new talent: smiling.

Have baby, will travel

Using a back carrier or sling accomplishes two goals: it gets a parent out of the house while at the same time keeping the baby snug and happy. It also frees up a parent's arms to do light tasks. These devices can be especially welcome to a new mum who feels out of shape. With her baby in a carrier, a mum can take a walk and get a little exercise. Meanwhile, the baby gets to see the outside world. Be sure to choose a carrier or sling that is right for your baby's weight and age, and follow the instructions so you use it safely.

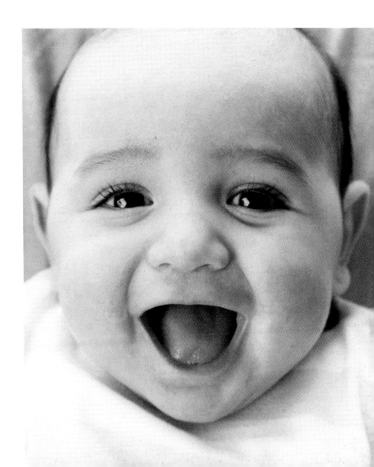

A happy baby
Learning new skills such as holding his or her head steady and grasping toys – and your fingers – will make your baby smile with delight.

Exploring at three to six months

Your baby's movements, which once seemed random and jerky, are becoming more orderly and purposeful. Now is a great time to create a childproof play space that will make it safe for your baby to explore his or her new world.

Improving coordination

During these months, your baby will learn to hold his or her head steady and sit with support. He or she will be able to open and close the hands that were once locked in tight fists. Tummy time remains important because your baby needs it to further improve head control and upper body strength. While on the floor, he or she will learn to prop themselves up – the first step towards exploring their new environment and rolling over.

A safe space for exploration

Exercise saucers and bouncing chairs, as well as other baby equipment, keep babies in one place, but they don't provide the kind of activity needed. Exercise saucers are fun and let the baby bounce, spin, and play with different toys. But they shouldn't be used for more than 30 minutes a day, broken into two or more brief sessions. If your child starts crying and seems bored, he or she probably is.

Avoid the temptation to let your baby use a walker with wheels (for information about these, see page 86). A safe play space is a better choice (see below for how to create such a space). In addition to being safe, the space should also be inviting and fun. To ensure this, place toys in reach, sit on the floor to play with your child, and make sure your baby has room to wiggle, squirm, and stretch.

Social butterflies

Babies seem to come alive socially during these months. They stare intently at faces and enjoy their first laughs. They enjoy being out and about, even if you are just going to the corner shop. Because they're more interactive and physically able, it opens up new possibilities for activities. Babies draw you in with a smile or a coo and are able to have extended play sessions. Playing can simply mean holding out a toy and letting your baby reach for it – even better if the baby is in your lap, where he or she can practise sitting up too.

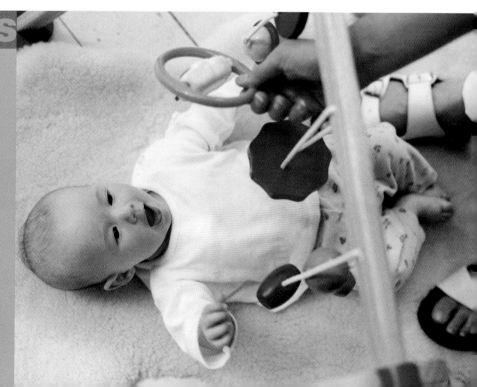

tips

A childproof play space

Creating a childproof space doesn't mean spending a lot of money. It simply means finding a room or part of a room and making it safe for the baby to explore – with supervision.
- Install stairgates to block entrances or staircases.
- Cover electrical sockets and tie up curtain cords.
- Put breakable items out of reach.
- Remove tables or other furniture that could tip over, and pad all the corners.

When the room is safe, let your baby move around, finding toys and other fun things to do.

Sitting and standing at six to nine months

Because babies are increasingly active at this age, parents have the opportunity to encourage the accomplishments they're so eager for their child to achieve, which include sitting without support and starting to stand up.

The balancing act

Being able to change positions is one of a baby's greatest achievements during these months. They can roll in both directions, sit without support, sit and pivot (without falling over), get from their tummy to a sitting position, and, finally, pull up to a stand. They also may have devised novel ways of transporting themselves where they want to go: rolling, scooting, or creeping. A parent can help a child work on balance in the sitting position by strategically placing objects within reach so the baby can practise this skill – and feel a sense of accomplishment when the desired toy is grabbed.

Standing up

When your child can support his or her weight, it's time to practise standing with support. Let your child lay on your lap or the floor and let him or her hold your hand and pull up to a stand. Once the child is good at that, he or she also might like to stand and bounce, so turn on some music and let the baby feel the beat. He or she also may be able to stand with support from the cot bars or sofa. Before you know it, your child will be doing this without any help.

Mind-body connection

Babies make huge cognitive strides during these months as they figure out the world around them. For instance, a baby learns how an object – or person – is still there even if partially covered. Place a blanket over a toy and voila! It's still there. That's why Peek-a-Boo is a great game for babies of this age. (See below for more games to play with your child.)

Your baby also starts to grasp cause and effect. Maybe you have found yourself trapped in this game: baby drops the toy, you give it back, and he or she drops it again. Or your baby may delight in hitting a wooden spoon against a saucepan. That's another example of cause and effect because your baby realizes that banging the pan makes a noise. It's satisfying because it's a way of demonstrating "I am here!"

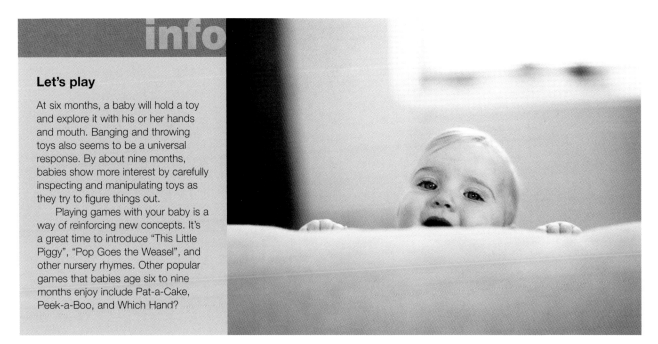

Let's play

At six months, a baby will hold a toy and explore it with his or her hands and mouth. Banging and throwing toys also seems to be a universal response. By about nine months, babies show more interest by carefully inspecting and manipulating toys as they try to figure things out.

Playing games with your baby is a way of reinforcing new concepts. It's a great time to introduce "This Little Piggy", "Pop Goes the Weasel", and other nursery rhymes. Other popular games that babies age six to nine months enjoy include Pat-a-Cake, Peek-a-Boo, and Which Hand?

On the move at nine to twelve months

During this last phase of their first year babies seem to be going somewhere all the time – up the stairs, under the table, from one end of the room to the other, pulling themselves up and along with whatever they can get their hands on.

Getting into trouble

Most babies at this age can scoot, creep, or crawl. They will pull up to a stand and "cruise" around using the furniture as support. Walking may be just around the corner for many of them. Parents can hold their baby's hands so the child can practise walking. Push-and-pull toys also can come in handy because they give a child something to hold on to, offering a bit of support. Many babies also love trying to climb the stairs – with a parent close by, of course. Trailing this busy person is a great workout for parents too.

Babies can get into trouble very quickly, even in the short amount of time it takes for a parent to answer the phone or check on dinner. So remember to keep stairgates closed and, when possible, close doors to those rooms that might contain hazards, such as the bathroom or kitchen. Also ensure that all sharp or dangerous objects are kept up high, well out of their reach, because babies will be sure to open all the cupboards at their level.

Because so much is off-limits, your baby will enjoy it if one of the floor-level cupboards is fair territory. Fill it with safe toys or household objects such as plastic containers. This also gives the baby something to do while adults are in the kitchen, preparing meals or doing other kitchen tasks.

While sometimes it seems your baby is just bent on making a mess, remember that he or she benefits from all this stimulating activity. Babies are learning critical skills and they're understandably determined to learn to move around and figure out how things work.

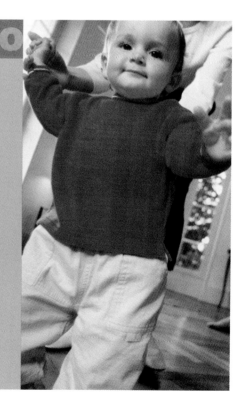

The baby who's not walking yet

While people look for babies to walk by age one, the truth is that most babies don't walk that early. As with other big achievements, such as sitting up, there's no one magic age that is associated with developing a skill. Rather, there's a range of months during which most children are expected to reach that milestone. The usual range for starting to walk is between nine and 16 months, but that doesn't mean some normal children won't walk a little later or take a few steps sooner.

It's also important to know that walking early isn't a sign of superior intelligence. Later walkers usually can look forward to being just as bright and physically active as their peers who walked sooner.

A child may be a late walker because his parents walked later. In extreme cases, such as in some foreign orphanages, a child may have been confined in a cot and didn't get the opportunity to develop the strength and skills necessary for walking. But sometimes a child who isn't walking by 18 months may have a medical condition. If you have any concerns about your child's development, discuss them with your doctor.

If your child has been growing and developing normally until this point, there is no cause to be concerned that your one-year-old hasn't taken his or her first step. It's just one more achievement to look forward to as your child enters the second year of life.

What's on the agenda?

It's true what people say about babies being more interested in the box and wrapping paper than in whatever gift the packaging held. Things around the house may interest babies as much as – or more than – any toy.

Between nine and 12 months, babies like big cardboard boxes they can stack or crawl through and crinkly paper they can crunch. When it's time to open the toy box, reach for balls and blocks. Roll or hand a ball to your baby, and demonstrate how to stack blocks, letting your child knock down your tower.

Books of all types will be of interest to your child. Fabric books and board books make it easy for babies to turn the pages. Look for books that have flaps to lift, textures to touch, and sounds to hear. When you run out of books to look at, visit the library for a fresh supply. It's a whole new place for your baby to explore.

Parents need to be vigilant
Close supervision, always important, takes on new significance now because babies can really get from one place to another in a flash.

Q: My ten-month-old baby isn't crawling. What should I do?

A: Crawling is a favourite infant milestone, but not every child crawls. This is no cause for alarm if your child has made steady progress in his or her motor development by rolling over, sitting, pulling up to stand, cruising, and so on. You may have noticed that prior to learning to walk a child devises some unique ways of getting around, including rolling, scooting on his or her bottom, or creeping.

While it's not a critical motor skill, here are some ways to encourage crawling in the older baby:

- Allow for tummy time so your baby is in the right position to practise crawling.
- Help your baby get into the crawling position on hands and knees.
- Position a favourite toy just out of reach and encourage your baby to move towards it.
- Limit the time your baby spends in pushchairs and cots so he or she has more opportunity to move.

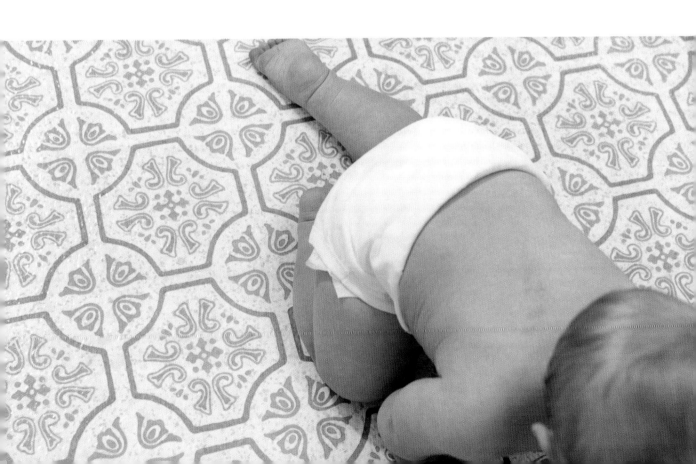

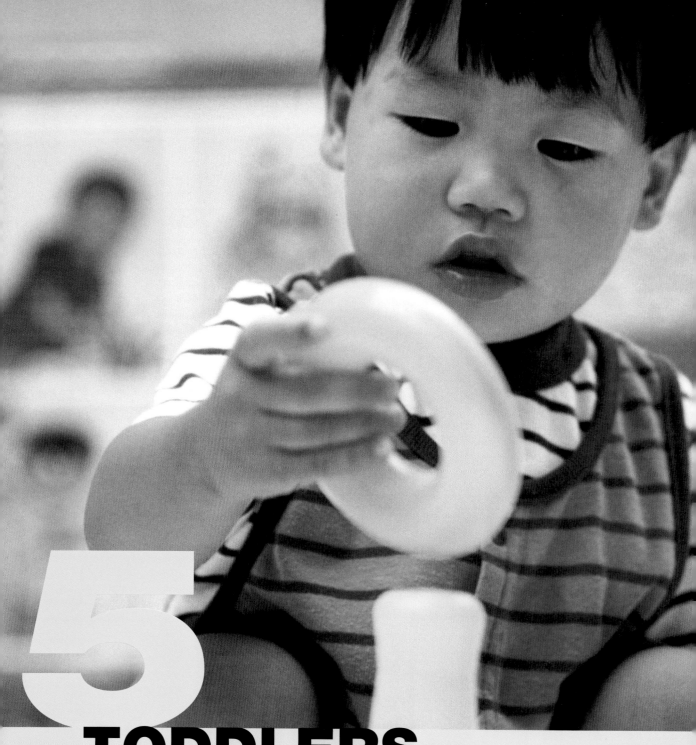

5 TODDLERS

Between the ages of one and three, children **walk away from babyhood** in search of independence. Parents should let them **have their independence** – in measured amounts – when it comes to eating and activity.

age 1–3

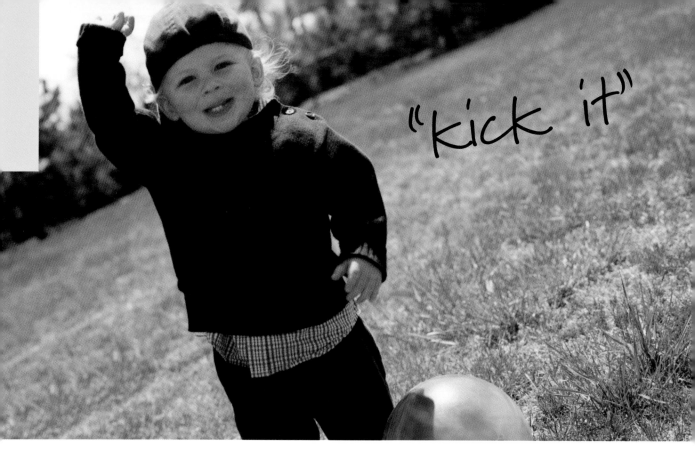

"kick it"

Toddlers on the move

Between the ages of one and three, children are both formidable and lovable. Toddlers push the limits – and their parents' buttons – as they try to figure out how to navigate the world.

Parents provide the structure

Toddlers want their independence and may express it loudly – it's during this period that the "terrible twos" can take hold. But they also don't want to stray too far from mum or dad, who are the source of security and safety. Parents can provide the right environment for their child by setting boundaries when it comes to eating and activity.

Parents should provide the kinds of foods that an active toddler needs. But anyone who has a child of this age knows how independent-minded they can be, so parents will have to work with their toddler and exert control in a crafty way. For instance, try presenting two healthy snacks and let your child choose which one to eat. In this way, your toddler will feel in control, but you will accomplish your goal of getting him or her to eat a nutritious snack – and without the usual battle.

Parents should also provide structure for physical activity. It's not difficult to get toddlers to be active – their high-energy style can wear a parent out – but toddlers need creative adults to help them channel all that energy into activities that are both fun, productive, and safe. A parent can fill the role of activity coordinator by leading a game of "Simon Says", playing catch, or helping the child sing action songs like "Head and Shoulders, Knees and Toes". Toddlers also need their parents to be there when it's time to stop exploring and settle in for a good night's sleep.

Toddlers are fussy eaters

A toddler may express his or her independence through eating – or not eating, as the case may be. Nearly all toddlers could be described as fussy eaters. Children of this age are famous for their reactions to new foods. They are naturally suspicious and, if they agree to try a spoonful, they may reject the new taste or texture. A toddler may also choose to play with food rather than eat it, or may want to eat only macaroni cheese for days. But because you choose the foods on your toddler's plate, you don't have to serve macaroni cheese every day. Instead, you can influence your child's food preferences by presenting a variety of nutritious foods to make up a healthy menu.

Feeding guidelines

What does this mean when deciding what to offer your toddler? Refer to the chart below to get an idea of what – and how much – your child should be eating. The number of servings per day is based on the Balanced Plate model (see page 40). The serving sizes are smaller than what is recommended for older children, with the exception of the dairy group. (Toddlers need at least two servings of dairy foods or 350ml/12floz of milk, which can be spread out over the course of a day.) The chart recommends the number of servings per day of each group. Keep in mind that younger toddlers may not eat this much at first.

Growing from baby to child

Babies grow at a lightning pace – 8cm (3 inches) or so every three months. The toddler, in contrast, grows at a much slower rate – only 8–13cm (3–5 inches) in an entire year. Growth slows markedly by 18–24 months. Pound for pound, a toddler actually needs fewer calories than an infant. This remains the case in the pre-school years and beyond.

Toddlers are in the midst of a transformation from baby to young child. During the toddler years, they will lose that "baby" look as they get leaner, stronger, and more active. It's also a period of amazing physical accomplishments as toddlers progress from barely walking to being able to run with agility by the age of three.

How much should **your toddler eat?**

Compared to older children, toddlers need fewer and smaller-sized servings from each of the basic food groups (the exception is fruits and vegetables, where the number of servings is the same). The chart below can be used as a guideline when feeding your toddler, but remember that each child is unique. Your GP can make specific recommendations for your child. Serving size may vary, and your child may eat more or less on any given day.

FOOD GROUP	DAILY SERVINGS	SIZE OF SERVING (12–24 MONTHS)	SIZE OF SERVING (24–36 MONTHS)
Carbohydrate foods	at least 4	¼–½ slice of bread; 2–4 tbsp cooked rice, pasta, or infant cereal	½–1 slice of bread; 4–8 tbsp cooked rice or pasta; 30g (1oz) breakfast cereal
Dairy foods	at least 2	175ml (6floz) milk or yogurt; 40g (1½oz) cheese	175ml (6floz) milk or yogurt; 40g (1½oz) cheese
Protein foods	1–2	1–2 tbsp or 15–30g (½–1oz) meat; 1 egg	30–55g (1–2oz) meat; 1 egg
Fruits	2–3	1 small banana, ½ apple or pear, 30ml (1floz) orange or apple juice, diluted	1 small banana, ½ apple or pear, 30ml (1floz) orange or apple juice, diluted
Vegetables	2–3	40g (1½oz) broccoli, carrots, sweetcorn, green beans, peas, or tomatoes	40g (1½oz) broccoli, carrots, sweetcorn, green beans, peas, or tomatoes

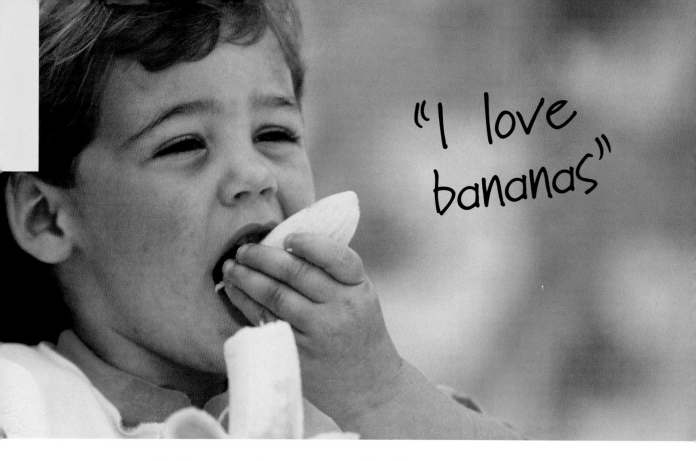

"I love bananas"

Nutrition for toddlers

Toddlers are beginning to discover what they like, and don't like, to eat – remember that it wasn't so long ago they were trying solids for the first time. Parents are in charge of providing healthy choices.

What toddlers need

In general, toddlers need about 1000–1200 calories a day, which they get in little bites and nibbles of food. From 12–24 months they are in transition from an infant diet, which is high in fat: by the age of two, a toddler should be getting no more than 35 percent of daily calories from fat.

Here's a breakdown of some of the important components in a toddler's diet and their needs. (See pages 34–39 for more information about these components.)

Protein: 14.5 grams a day.

Calcium: 350 milligrams a day, due to the high requirement during this period of rapid growth and development.

Iron: 6.9 milligrams a day.

Fibre: There are no official recommendations for fibre intake in children, but they should have proportionally less than the 18 grams a day recommended for adults. A high-fibre diet is bulky and young children have small appetites.

Milk matters

An important part of a toddler's diet, milk provides calcium and vitamin D to help build strong bones. Children under age two should have whole milk to help provide the dietary fats they need for normal growth and brain development. After age two, most kids can switch to semi-skimmed milk, providing they are eating a good variety of family foods. Skimmed milk should not be introduced until after age five.

Some kids initially reject cow's milk because it doesn't taste like the familiar breast milk or formula. If your child is around 12 months of age and having this difficulty, mix whole milk with some formula or breast milk. Gradually adjust the mixture over time so it becomes 100-percent cow's milk.

Meeting iron requirements

After 12 months of age, toddlers are at risk of iron deficiency because they no longer drink iron-fortified formula and may not be eating iron-fortified infant cereal or enough other iron-containing foods to make up the difference. Drinking a lot of cow's milk (more than 600ml/1 pint every day) can also put a young child at risk of developing iron deficiency. Here's why:

- Cow's milk is low in iron.
- Toddlers who drink a lot of cow's milk may be less hungry and less likely to eat iron-rich foods.
- Milk decreases the absorption of iron and can also irritate the lining of the intestine, causing small amounts of bleeding and the gradual loss of iron in the stool.

Iron deficiency can affect a child's growth and may lead to learning and behavioural problems. And it can progress to anaemia, which is a decreased number of red blood cells in a person's body. Iron is needed to make red blood cells, which carry oxygen throughout the body. Without enough iron and red blood cells, the body's tissues and organs get less oxygen and don't function as well.

To help prevent iron deficiency:

- Limit your toddler's milk intake to no more than 600ml (1 pint) a day.
- Increase iron-rich foods in your child's diet (see page 157 for a list of these foods).
- Serve iron-fortified cereal until your child is 18–24 months of age.

Talk to your doctor if your child drinks a lot of cow's milk or you are concerned that he or she is not eating a balanced diet. Many toddlers are checked for iron-deficiency anaemia. A child who has anaemia will probably need to take an iron supplement, but never give your child a vitamin or mineral supplement without first discussing it with the doctor.

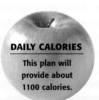

DAILY CALORIES
This plan will provide about 1100 calories.

One-day menu planner **for toddlers**

Serving sizes for most foods in a toddler's diet will vary according to the child's age and appetite. Milk – and water – are the best drinks to serve between meals. Sweetened drinks, including diluted fruit juice, should only be consumed with meals, to reduce the risk of dental caries.

breakfast
- small glass of apple juice diluted with water
- fortified cereal with milk

FOOD GROUP	SERVINGS
carbs	1
dairy	0
protein	0
fruits	1
vegetables	0

snack
- 1 small banana
- 175ml (6floz) milk

FOOD GROUP	SERVINGS
carbs	0
dairy	1
protein	0
fruits	1
vegetables	0

lunch
- small glass of apple juice diluted with water
- 1 scrambled or boiled egg with toast
- small bunch of grapes

FOOD GROUP	SERVINGS
carbs	1 1/2
dairy	0
protein	1
fruits	2
vegetables	0

snack
- 1 breadstick with hummus
- few carrot sticks

FOOD GROUP	SERVINGS
carbs	1/2
dairy	0
protein	0
fruits	0
vegetables	1

tea
- tuna and sweetcorn with pasta
- 1 small pot fromage frais

FOOD GROUP	SERVINGS
carbs	1
dairy	1
protein	1
fruits	0
vegetables	1

bedtime
- 175ml (6floz) milk

FOOD GROUP	SERVINGS
carbs	0
dairy	1
protein	0
fruits	0
vegetables	0

Food preferences at 12–24 months

Young toddlers become experts at eating as they come to accept new tastes and textures and feed themselves with increasing proficiency. For the parent it is a golden opportunity to influence what a child chooses to eat for years to come.

Adjusting to a changing menu

Just when you had the routine mastered, your toddler's diet is changing. Bottles and baby food are on their way out. Milk and more family food are on the way in. But none of these changes occurs overnight, so parents can help toddlers ease into the new eating routine. Use the chart on page 95 and your own judgement to make sure your child is satisfied and getting adequate nutrition. Parents of toddlers have another important job: to help kids develop a taste for healthy food. Children are more likely to reject nutritious foods if they don't try them early in life. If given the easy option of sweets, biscuits, chocolate, and ice cream, children will often tend to choose these foods over healthier fare later on.

If children don't like a food, they won't eat it – no rocket science there. But don't be discouraged if your toddler doesn't like a food the first time you offer it. Children of this age are naturally slow to accept new tastes and textures, and you may have to present the food ten or more times before they'll finally give it a try.

If, for example, your toddler doesn't like green beans the first time round, don't stop serving them. Just keep reintroducing the beans without nagging or forcing your child to eat them. Simply make small portions of the food available so the child can give them another try. And be sure you're setting a good example by eating the food yourself! Serve nutritious foods that you like so your child will see you enjoying what you're asking them to eat.

Letting your child not eat

While the goal may be to broaden a child's palate, a parent also needs to relinquish a certain amount of control to the child – even at this young age. A parent's role is to present

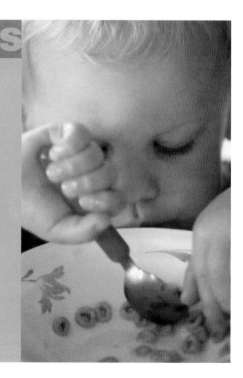

tips

Learning to eat like big kids

Toddlers are beginning to eat more independently – first with their fingers and then using utensils to feed themselves. This transition can be messy as toddlers are notoriously sloppy eaters, but if they have the opportunity to experiment they will improve their skills over time.

Finger foods

While fostering independent eating, parents should watch out for choking risk by serving finger foods that are easy to chew and cut into small pieces. Stay with your child if giving hard fruit and vegetables, such as raw carrots and apple slices. Avoid whole nuts.

Minimizing the mess

Here are some suggestions to help you limit the mess caused by your toddler's sloppy eating:

- Use appropriate-size utensils.
- Place a plastic mat on the floor under the high chair.
- Use large plastic bibs or bibs with pockets.
- Serve drinks in feeder cups.
- Have wet facecloths to hand to wipe your child's hands and face after the meal.
- If your child will be eating when out and about, bring a wet facecloth or disposable wipes, a bib, and a change of clothes so you're prepared for anything!

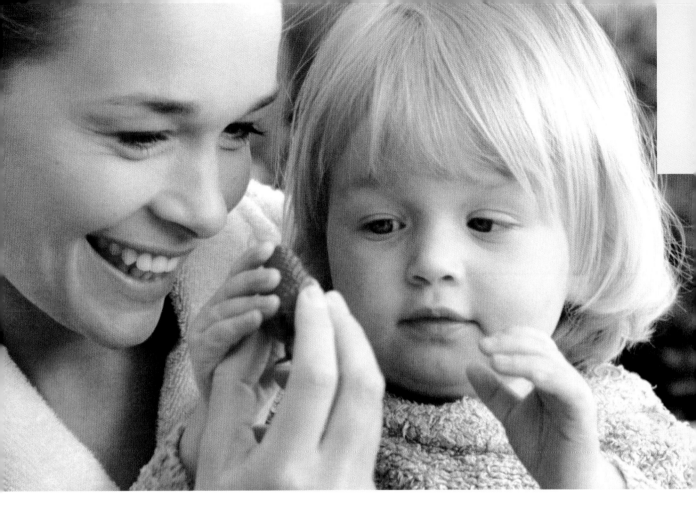

healthy foods and let the child decide which ones to eat – or whether to eat at all. Be alert to what your toddler is saying through his or her actions. A child who is playing with his or her food may be telling you he or she is full.

Allowing a child to skip a meal is a difficult concept because many of us were raised to eat everything on our plates and not waste food. But children should be allowed to respond to their own hunger cues – a vital skill for maintaining a healthy weight. That means eating when hungry, and sometimes not eating, even if it's time for Sunday lunch.

Pushing food on a child who's not hungry may dull the internal cues that help a child know when he or she is full. But that doesn't mean that it's practical or advisable for the child to eat on demand all day long. That's why structured meals and snack times are important. Your child will come to expect that food will be available during certain times of the day. At those times your child can decide whether to eat, as

Good things to eat
Use this golden opportunity to broaden a child's palate by exposing your toddler to a wide range of healthy foods, from fruits and vegetables to whole grains.

well as which foods to eat and how much of them to eat. If the child chooses not to eat anything at all, simply offer food again at the next meal or snack.

Practising feeding skills

At mealtime, let your child finger feed and practise using utensils, a skill typically learned at 15–18 months. Give your child many opportunities to do these things. Early on, make sure the child isn't too hungry or the experience may lead to frustration. During this transition, jump in and help feed your child when necessary, but try to pay attention to the child's hunger cues and note signs that he or she is full. You can always offer more if your child still seems hungry, but you can't take the food back if you've overfed your child.

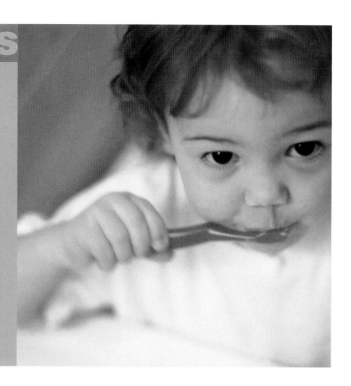

tips

Toddler teeth need cleaning

It's important to keep a toddler's teeth clean, to reduce plaque and the risk of cavities. While older toddlers may be able to brush on their own with supervision, they all still need mum or dad to do some proper brushing.

- Clean your toddler's teeth twice a day, preferably after breakfast and before bed.
- Use a child-sized toothbrush with soft bristles.
- Until age two use a toothpaste specially formulated for children (as these pastes taste good, encourage your child to spit them out rather than swallow). After age two you can switch to adult toothpaste but use only a pea-sized amount.
- Take care to brush all tooth surfaces to remove plaque and debris. Don't forget behind the teeth as well as the gums and tongue.
- To prevent dental caries, limit sugary snacks and don't allow your child (of any age) to sip on juice or milk for extended periods.

When you're controlling the fork or spoon, resist the urge to slip in one more bite. And as your toddler gets the hang of eating, step back and let your child take over.

Little and often

Many toddlers need to eat often – as much as six times a day, including three meals and three snacks. Keep this in mind as you establish a pattern of meal and snacks. And remember that the schedule only establishes the times that you will present food to your toddler. Your child may not take every opportunity to eat.

Try to avoid offering snacks just before mealtimes or pacifying a hungry child with a cup of milk or water right before a meal. Eating and drinking just before meals can diminish appetite and decrease your child's willingness to try the new food you are offering at mealtimes.

When to stop bottlefeeding

Around 12 months of age your child will be switching from breast milk or formula to cow's milk. By then most children have learned to drink from a feeder cup – after the age of six months a baby can be encouraged to start trying the cup – so it can be a natural transition from formula in a bottle

to milk in a cup. If you are breastfeeding, only offer milk in a feeder cup and avoid the bottle habit altogether. By 12–18 months of age children should have 350–600ml (12–20floz) of milk per day. Drinking more milk than this can get in the way of eating a balanced diet and may also put the child at risk for iron deficiency. (For more information about iron deficiency, see page 97.)

Some young toddlers may be attached to the bottle as a source of comfort. Practically speaking, it's best to stop giving the bottle sooner rather than later because, over time, kids get increasingly resistant to giving it up and will have more to say in the matter.

Instead of cutting out bottles all at once, gradually eliminate them from the feeding schedule, starting with mealtime. Offer cow's milk from a cup after your child has begun the meal. Generally, the nighttime bottle is the last to go because it is part of the bedtime routine. If this is the case, let your child have a cup of milk with his or her evening snack and continue with the rest of your nighttime ritual (bath, bedtime story, teeth cleaning, etc). No matter how old the child is, no child should go to bed with a bottle because it can cause serious tooth decay. (See above for information about looking after your toddler's teeth.)

Eating by themselves at 24–36 months

The older toddler's desire for independence and control is intense. It's no wonder this age is called the "terrible twos". By anticipating problems and offering choices, you can teach your child which behaviours will yield positive results and which ones won't.

Conflict at mealtimes

When a two-year-old doesn't get what he or she wants, be prepared for a major tantrum. Although this behaviour is challenging, to say the least, it has a purpose. Toddlers are learning how to navigate the world, communicate in it, and figure out how to exert control over aspects of their lives. Although toddlers actually have control over very little, they are starting to master eating and using the toilet. A child can't – and shouldn't – be forced to do either one of these.

Because older toddlers often use eating to express their independence, food and mealtimes can cause conflict. You want your child to eat the vegetables on his or her plate; the child drops them on to the floor. You want him or her to eat the meal you prepared for the family; the child is clamouring for chicken nuggets, which is the only food he or she is willing to eat. A well-meaning parent's impulse may be to pick up the spoon and start feeding the child the healthy food on the plate. You also might start "talking up" those nutritious foods, telling the child how big and strong broccoli will make him or her. Or you might start bargaining: "Well, if you eat three more bites of chicken, I'll give you a biscuit." The problem is, none of those tactics work in the long run.

Playing with their food
Toddlers are explorers in all realms, including the food on their plate or in their bowl. Finger feeding allows them to investigate the feel of the food before they eat it.

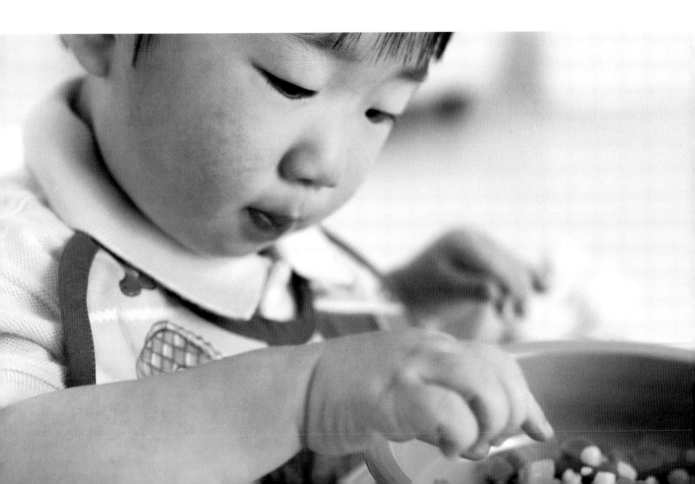

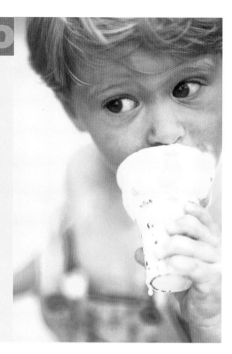

Don't use food as a reward

During the toddler years, avoid the temptation to reward a toddler with food, particularly with sweets and biscuits. Toddlers respond to positive reinforcement and food rewards can be very powerful. But there's a big downside to using food as an incentive: it can start a pattern of unhealthy eating behaviour. Also, if the child is offered a biscuit, not a piece of fruit, for good behaviour, the child may get the message that sweets are more valuable than other, more nutritious foods.

Instead of rewarding your child with food, take a deep breath and try to find another solution.

- If your child appears to be bored, try to get him or her interested in a toy or game.
- If your child wants some of your time, take a few moments and give him or her a little attention.
- If your child is hungry, provide a healthy snack.
- If your child needs a reward for a job well done, offer a big hug instead of a sugary treat.

As with all toddler behaviour, consistency is key, so both parents and all carers should adopt the same tactics. If this is not done, the toddler might get confused, or learn which parent to ask for a snack.

Parents taking over

You may think that not letting your child feed himself or herself is for the child's own good, but it takes away control that rightfully belongs to a child of this age. Children need to decide whether to eat, what they will eat, and how much to eat – this is how they are going to learn to recognize their own internal cues that tell them when they are hungry and when they're full. Just as important, toddlers need to learn and practise the mechanics of feeding themselves.

Talking up certain foods

Who hasn't used the line about spinach making you strong? But this cajoling approach may build dislike for the healthy food rather than increase acceptance. By the same token, forbidding less nutritious foods makes them more desirable. This doesn't mean you shouldn't teach your child about the benefits of healthy foods, but don't push too much by celebrating every bite of spinach or broccoli your toddler eats or disapproving when he or she refuses.

Making deals

Because older toddlers need to decide for themselves if they are hungry, it's not a good idea to bribe them into eating a certain amount of food. It creates an unnecessary power struggle at the table as the bargaining gets more intense. This tactic can lead to conflict when the child whines about reducing the number of bites or refuses to eat any more food. It is a battle you will not win. Worse yet, the child learns to use food as a bargaining ploy.

For some children, mealtime becomes a negotiation session from the very start, and parents have been using dessert as an incentive for decades. But this doesn't encourage healthy eating. Instead it creates the impression that "treats" are more valuable than mealtime food. Sweet foods are not essential to your child's diet and it is not a deprivation to avoid serving them during the toddler years.

If your child has tried sweets and demands them, it's time to stop buying them. As a parent, you control which foods are in the house and you decide which ones to serve to your child. If you do not regularly buy sweets and less nutritious snack foods, your child won't see them, clamour for them, and feel angry when you do not oblige.

If your toddler asks for sweets, simply say, "We don't have any". Then present the child with two healthy snack alternatives and let him or her choose one. Even if the child mourns the loss of the sweets, he or she will still feel a sense of control by getting to make the decision about which of the healthy snacks to eat.

How to get a toddler to eat well

In addition to everything else toddlers are learning, they are also learning how to get what they want. Parents need to stand firm. Doing so will limit clashes and encourage healthy eating. Here are some additional guidelines.

- Stock the cupboards with healthy foods: Toddlers aren't going to run out to the shop for a packet of crisps; they'll eat what's served to them and ask for what they know is in the cupboard.
- Serve right-sized portions: Parents often overestimate how much food a child should eat. Especially with foods that aren't yet favourites, a couple of tablespoons is a good portion to start with. Small portions are less overwhelming for a child, while bigger portions may encourage overeating.
- Offer variety no matter what: If a child is stuck on one food, a parent might feel forced to serve that food every day so the child eats something. But eventually the child may tire of that food – and then what? In addition, you're missing an opportunity to introduce new foods and increase the number of foods your child is willing to eat. It's a good idea to continue offering a variety of foods even if your child rejects them repeatedly. Your toddler may surprise you one day. Most food fads don't last long if parents don't accommodate them. Children won't starve and they will learn to be more flexible rather than go hungry.

Q: My child will only eat food that is white. Should I force him to try other foods?

A: No, don't force him, but continue offering a variety of foods even if he often rejects them. Eating can be an emotional issue, so try to keep a cool head and be smart about the strategies you employ. Help him establish healthy preferences that will serve him well through the years. Know that most healthy kids eat enough food to grow and develop normally, but also trust your instincts if you're concerned your child isn't eating enough or failing to eat enough healthy foods. Talk with your child's doctor or health visitor about your concerns. Going over your child's growth chart is a good way to make sure he is staying on track. Most toddlers don't need a multivitamin, but your doctor may recommend it if your child is a particularly fussy eater.

- Have family meals together: Children eat a more nutritious diet, with more fruits and vegetables, when they regularly have family meals.
- Create positive peer pressure: Toddlers are more likely to eat fruits and vegetables if they see their peers eating them, so look for opportunities where your child can eat healthily with friends, at home or at playgroups.

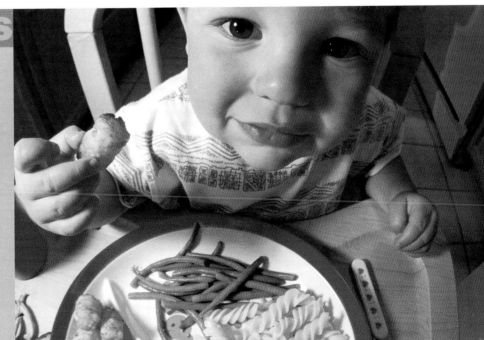

tips

Helping your toddler learn to eat at mealtimes

- Set your toddler's place at the family table – it's good for kids of this age to see their parents and siblings eating together and eating the right foods.
- Present a variety of foods, including some established favourites and some new foods.
- Serve small portions.
- Cut food into small pieces.
- Serve the drink after the child has started eating.
- Talk about something other than what the child is (or isn't) eating.

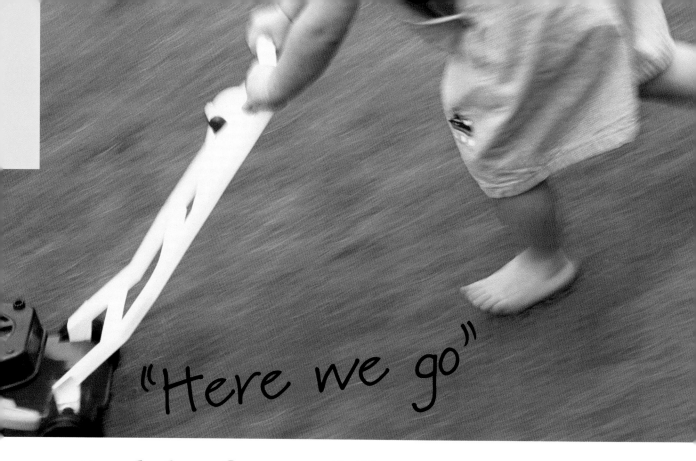

"Here we go"

Activity for toddlers

Toddlers have reason to be proud of their accomplishments, such as walking, running, and climbing. Over these years they master basic skills as they gain muscle control, balance, and coordination.

Physical skills to learn

Each new skill mastered allows a toddler to progress to the next one, building on a foundation that one day will enable him or her to perform more complicated physical tasks, such as skipping rope, kicking a ball, or turning a cartwheel. For a toddler, those days of turning cartwheels can't come soon enough. Children in this age range want to do more than they may be physically capable of doing. This can be a powerful motivator that drives them to keep trying until they acquire a new skill, no matter what it takes.

That's not to say that toddlers can do it alone. They need their parents to support them as they make progress. Here are some ways you can help your child.

- Know which physical skills your child is working on now and which ones will come later. (See the developing skills chart, opposite.)
- Provide opportunities for the child to be physically active.
- Choose activities the whole family can enjoy.
- Keep the child safe during all forms of activity.
- Minimize sedentary activities such as watching TV.

The more opportunities a parent provides, the more active the child will be. Take advantage of your toddler's natural desire to keep moving. Even at this early age a child is establishing patterns of activity that set the stage for the rest of childhood. If a toddler is inactive at three, there's a good chance that child will remain inactive later in life.

Developing **skills**

Playing and learning are completely enmeshed for toddlers, so acquiring the long list of skills below should be fun and games for them. Parents should give toddlers many opportunities to practise their developing skills – and provide a lot of supervision so they stay safe while they learn. In addition to these physical accomplishments, toddlers are developing in other ways. Provide opportunities for your child to explore, ask questions, use his or her imagination, and practise skills such as stacking blocks or colouring.

EARLY TODDLER SKILLS (12–24 MONTHS)

- walks independently
- pulls toys while walking
- carries toys while walking
- stoops and gets back up
- begins to run
- kicks a ball
- holds handrail up/down stairs
- walks backwards

OLDER TODDLER SKILLS (24–36 MONTHS)

- balances one to two seconds on one foot
- climbs well
- throws ball overhand
- bends over easily without falling
- runs and jumps well
- kicks ball forwards
- alternates feet up and down stairs
- pedals tricycle

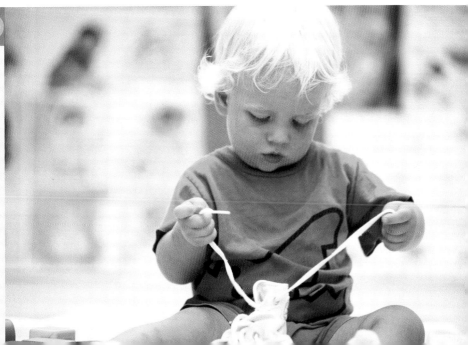

info

Walking shoes

Going barefoot indoors is fine when toddlers are learning to walk. Outdoors, though, shoes are needed. The shoes won't help your child walk, but they will protect tender feet from injury. Choose comfortable trainers or shoes that fit well and support the feet, instead of those big, clomping, white baby shoes that just get in the way.

A toddler's shoes should:
- have easily bendable soles;
- be flexible enough to allow foot and ankle movement;
- fit well enough that they don't slip and cause tripping.

How much **activity is enough?**

A good guideline is that toddlers should get 30 minutes or more a day of physical activity, such as playing on a playground, going for a walk, or taking a music and movement class. In addition, toddlers should get at least 60 minutes of free play when they can explore and play with toys.

Though it can be a workout for their parents and carers, toddlers ought to be moving most of their waking day. Children in this age range shouldn't stay inactive for prolonged periods of time – no longer than 60 minutes unless they're sleeping. To achieve this, avoid TV-watching or long stints in high chairs, in favour of free time down on the floor, so your toddler can move around.

	PHYSICAL ACTIVITY	FREE PLAY
Younger toddlers (12–24 months)	● listening to music and dancing together ● holding your child's hands while he or she jumps ● exploring the garden or playground together ● climbing stairs and using climbing equipment, with supervision	● using push-and-pull toys (vehicles, carts to load and unload, musical boxes) ● imitating animals or adults at work (making dinner, using tools) ● playing with shape sorters and other floor toys
Older toddlers (24–36 months)	● playing at the playground or in the garden together ● playing follow the leader, "Ring-a-ring-o-roses", and other similar games ● playing ball ● taking a music and movement or tumbling class for toddlers ● exercising together (see the suggested activities opposite)	● enjoying imaginative play (playing with toy cars, making play figures talk, caring for a doll) ● building with blocks ● drawing with crayons

Limit TV time

When caring for a toddler at home, there are so many hours to fill that a parent or other carer may be tempted to turn to passive activities such as watching TV. But limiting television is a very good way to help keep your child physically active. TV is not recommended at all for children under age two. Those suggested guidelines relax for older toddlers, but there's really no reason why your child must watch any TV at all. A toddler will get much more out of playing with a shape sorter, swinging on a swing, or hearing a book read by a caring adult. Even educational programmes aren't as enriching as real-life activities, such as working out how a toy functions or playing games and singing songs together.

If you choose to allow some TV time for your older toddler, try to limit it to a maximum of one to two hours of quality children's programmes per day. If possible, choose non-commercial television because commercial TV exposes children to food advertising that often pushes low-nutrient snack foods and drinks. Another option is age-appropriate videos, especially those that invite the child to play along.

Provide a safe environment

Wherever a toddler is being active, the play area must be safe. At home, use gates and other safety equipment to make at least one room in the house safe enough for a toddler to explore. Away from home, look for childcare

Q: My toddler wants to watch videos all the time. What should I do?

A: Children like repetition, which can lead to repeated requests to watch the same video over and over again. A toddler may be very insistent and even throw a tantrum if the desired film or programme isn't played on demand. Remember that you, the parent, are in charge. You can say "No" in a matter of fact way and direct your child to a different activity. Very few parents can claim that they have not used a video or DVD to keep a toddler occupied for a while. But try not to use the TV as a babysitter or a replacement for your time and attention. Even if it means delaying dinner by 15 minutes, take a little time in the evening to reconnect with your child, especially if you've been away from him or her all day. Toddlers are time-consuming little people because they need so much supervision, direction, and attention. But your efforts will help them learn to play independently and keep them from getting hooked on TV. Stick to your guns, and the next time your child wants to watch the video offer alternatives, such as colouring or doing puzzles together.

facilities and playgrounds that have newer, high-quality equipment that's not too big or challenging for your toddler. Also ask about whether children are separated by age – a practice that helps prevent injuries.

But no matter how "safe" the environment, there's no substitute for supervision. Many toddlers seem to subscribe to the "no fear" philosophy and may climb to the top of the monkey bars without reservation. Close supervision is important because, even as they show improving skills, toddlers lack sufficient balance, coordination, and judgement.

Activity away from home

If your toddler spends time with a childminder or at a nursery, it's important to investigate how much activity the children get on a regular basis.

- Do they go outside most days?
- Is there a schedule of activities that they adhere to?
- Do they watch videos or TV on a regular basis?

Another option is a playgroup, which is a great way to get children together for some active time. A playgroup is also a welcome change of pace for stay-at-home parents, who benefit from the social time with other mums and dads.

The parents could plan some time for structured group activities such as playing a game, and let the kids do their own thing for some of the time. Meeting at a playground or large, indoor space is ideal.

If you've ever seen a group of toddlers playing, they don't seem to be interacting as much as older children. Still, be assured they enjoy this time together. Eventually they will start playing in a more cooperative way.

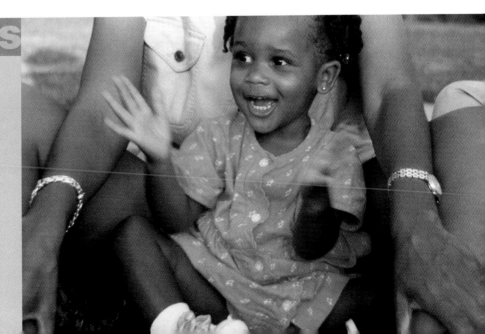

tips

Physical activities for parents and older toddlers

- Walk like a penguin, hop like a frog, or imitate other animals.
- Sit facing each other and hold hands. Rock back and forth, and sing "Row, Row, Row Your Boat".
- Bend at the waist and touch the ground. Walk your hands forwards and inch along like a caterpillar.
- Sit on the ground and let your child step over your legs, or make a bridge with your body and let your child crawl under.

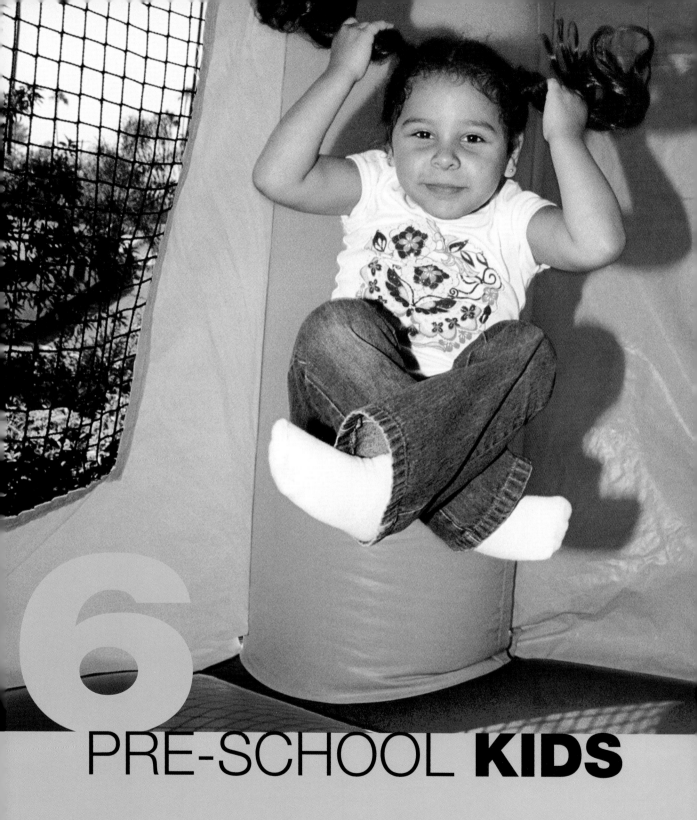

6

PRE-SCHOOL **KIDS**

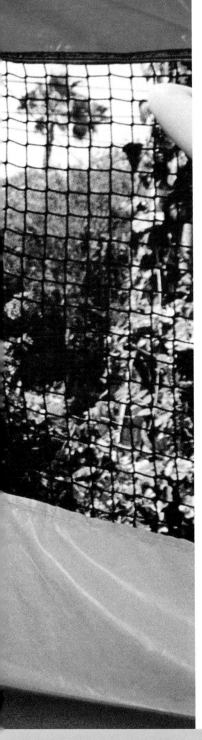

Is your pre-school child ready to **learn and grow**? You can help make this possible by **serving nutritious foods**, encouraging lots of physical activity, and helping your child get **ready for primary school**.

age 3-5

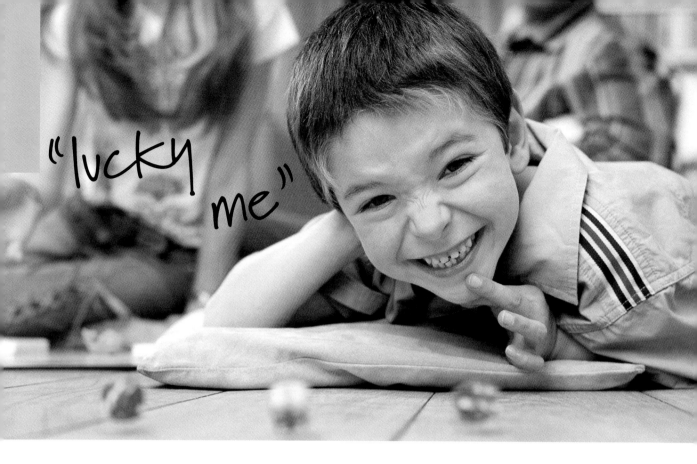

"lucky me"

Taking their place in the world

The pre-school years are a time of transition, when children become less dependent on parents and increasingly reliant on themselves. But as they idolize adults they're eager to please.

Emerging as individuals

Between the ages of three and five, children will start to move from a magical world to the real one, where the moon is made of moon rocks instead of green cheese. As pre-school children become more rational thinkers, they can better follow rules and instructions. They also will begin to understand the concept of consequences – another change that prepares them for the road ahead.

During the pre-school years, your child will emerge as an individual. No longer a toddler, he or she is less likely to throw a tantrum and should be more likely to cooperate – children of this age want to please their parents. And your child will want to be involved in whatever is going on, whether it's playing a game with older siblings or helping a parent do the household tasks or prepare dinner.

Inquisitive and opinionated

Pre-school children still get frustrated and they are still learning how to behave. However, they can communicate more effectively now. They are keenly aware of the world and are by nature inquisitive. Their drive to discover is evident in the many questions they ask their parents.

● What is that bug?
● Why is ice cold?

- Why do I have to wear shoes?
- Where does the sun go at night?

Children learn by asking questions and parents should try to answer them. One great place to talk is around the family dinner table. Through conversation, children will acquire language skills that help get them ready to learn at school.

In addition to talking, children like listening, especially to a story being read. Now that your child is older, try to involve him or her more in the reading. Here are some ideas:

- Ask your child to "read" you a story, turning the pages of a book and telling you what's happening.
- Stop and ask questions like "Where is Goldilocks going?" or "What do you think will happen next?"
- Ask your child to act out parts of the story.
- Encourage your child to create a picture about the story you've read. Most pre-school kids enjoy colouring, cutting (with child-safe scissors), pasting, and painting. Display your child's artwork and say how much you like it.

While pre-school children are people-pleasers, they also can be quite opinionated. They want to be heard. Whether it's a new food on their plate or their first swimming lesson, they will tell you – in no uncertain terms – if they liked it or not. But no matter how independent or outspoken they are, children of this age still need an adult to make most decisions. By limiting TV and computer time, parents can help lead their children towards becoming more physically active. Adults also guide their children towards better nutrition when they buy and serve healthy foods and drinks.

Learning how to be fit and healthy

The give-and-take of communication creates opportunities for parents. Whether it's playing or eating, pre-school kids want to do it themselves, but they are willing to learn from mum and dad. It's a great time to teach them about healthy food choices and how to be active in new and exciting ways.

At this age they are old enough to begin understanding the concept of being full, known as satiety. Children who stop eating when they feel full are less likely to become overweight. Most children naturally know if they are hungry or full and they can use these cues to properly control their food intake. Children who are encouraged to ignore these cues may learn to override this internal control mechanism.

A balanced diet gives children the nutrients necessary for optimal growth and development, and the energy for the exploration they want to do. Physical activity encourages children to develop muscle strength and endurance and to improve their motor skills. Through eating properly and playing a lot, pre-school children can maintain a healthy weight and be full of energy as they get ready for the next big step in their young lives: primary school.

tips

How does my garden grow?

Gardening can introduce children to nature and get them interested in healthy food. And, as you know if you've cared for a garden, it's good exercise. Here's how to cultivate your child's green thumb.

- Buy child-size garden tools, such as a rake and watering can, for your child. Larger tools can be difficult to use and frustrating for a small child.
- Consider starting out with seeds instead of young plants – children enjoy watching them germinate and grow. Pick seeds that are easy to care for and produce quick results, so children can see the fruits of their labour soon. Green beans, cucumbers, and pumpkins are good choices, as

are sunflowers, zinnias, and marigolds. Carrots take a while to germinate, but are fun to pull out of the ground.

- Let your child play a key role by helping you decide what to plant in the garden and helping you plant the seeds or seedlings. You also might turn over a small section to the child, who can choose to plant something there or just dig in the dirt.
- Keep your little gardener safe by avoiding the use of pesticides and other chemicals.
- In summer, make sure your child wears a hat and apply sun cream with a high sun protection factor (SPF). Also use a child-safe insect-repellant, if necessary.

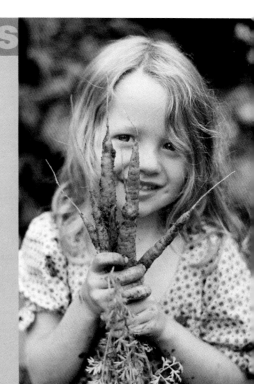

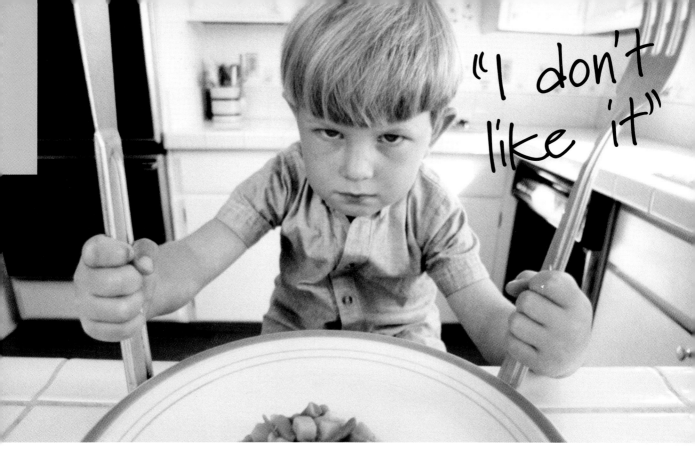

"I don't like it"

Nutrition for pre-school kids

Many food preferences are already established by the pre-school years, but parents still hold a lot of sway and it's a good time to introduce new foods to your children.

What pre-school kids need

Growth is slow and steady for pre-school children, whose daily needs increase by about 100 calories a year between the ages of two and five. During these years children typically eat 1200–1600 calories a day, depending on their activity level. Here are some key nutrients and guidelines for how much your child should have each day (see pages 34–39 for more information about these nutrients).

Protein: between 14 and 20 grams a day.

Fibre: There are no official recommendations for fibre intake, but a good guideline is about 6 grams a day.

Calcium: requirements increase during these years – from 350 milligrams a day to 450 milligrams by the time a child is four. The calcium requirement can be a challenge if your child doesn't like milk. But calcium can be found in other dairy foods, such as cheese and yogurt, as well as in calcium-fortified foods.

Iron: about 6 milligrams a day.

The parents' role

At a parent's request, a pre-school child may be willing to try new foods – especially if mum and dad are eating the same thing. In addition to watching what you eat your child learns other lessons at the family table, including how to act at mealtime. You can expect more of a pre-school child than a toddler, but don't expect perfection. Work on teaching your

Q: **My four-year-old just will not try new foods. I'm at my wits' end. Should I give up?**

A: Research shows it may take as many as ten tries before a child accepts a new food. So if your child doesn't seem to like a new food, don't give up. Never force or bribe a child to eat, and don't make a big issue out of it if your child chooses not to eat. By presenting the new food over and over again, you increase the chances your child will try it. Eventually, your child may decide to try the food and might even like it!

child proper use of utensils, where the napkin goes, sitting up straight at the table – and how to say "No, thank you" rather than "Yuck!"

Guiding a child's eating habits is delicate work. You want to encourage your child to make good choices but without pestering. You should take charge by presenting mostly healthy foods, but you don't want to teach your child that certain foods are "bad". You want your child to eat enough nutritious food, but you don't want to start negotiating how many bites of dinner must be eaten to get dessert. These approaches don't work and may even make it more likely that a child will eat too many calories.

Parents can take these steps to encourage a well-rounded diet:
- Continue offering a variety of foods, even ones the child has rejected in the past.
- Keep healthy foods in the house and limit the availability of high-calorie, low-nutrient foods.
- Involve children in meal preparation – for example, let them tear lettuce for a salad or help lay the table.
- Create a structure for daily meals and snacks so the child doesn't graze all day long.
- Have regular family meals and make them pleasant times for the whole family to get together.
- Set a good example by eating a nutritious diet yourself.

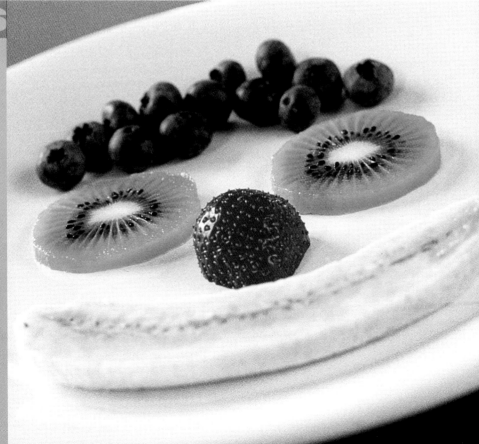

tips

Eye appeal

To tempt a young child, here are some ideas for making healthy foods look good and fun to eat.

Food faces Make facial features by arranging fruits or vegetables on a plate, or on a slice of bread or a bagel half spread with peanut butter or cream cheese. Try blueberry hair, kiwi fruit eyes, a strawberry nose, and a banana smile.

Flower power Arrange apple slices to make flower petals. Use a few slices of kiwi fruit for the centres.

Cute cut-outs Use biscuit cutters to fashion sandwiches or slices of cheese into hearts, stars, and favourite animal shapes.

Pretty pancakes Make Scotch pancake (drop scone) batter and cook in shaped moulds on the pan.

Is your child really hungry?

Parents need to talk to children about what it means to be hungry and what it means to be full. Most of us are born with the ability to gauge our body's need for food, but over time we can learn to ignore these signals, which may contribute to weight gain. Not surprisingly, kids who don't recognize when they're full are more likely to be overweight.

Around the pre-school years, many children start to use the word "hungry" to express other feelings, such as boredom, loneliness, sadness, and other emotions they don't understand or are unable to name. Using food to relieve sadness, for instance, will establish the connection between food and feelings other than hunger. Over time that can be increasingly difficult to undo. And it won't address the underlying reason for the sadness either.

If your child complains of hunger, take a minute to gently probe and make sure that's what's really going on. When your child says, "I'm hungry", ask "What have you been doing?" or "Would you like me to play with you for a while?"

If your child quickly forgets about a snack, you'll know that he or she was in search of your attention or just looking for something to do.

It's just as important to avoid inadvertently encouraging your child to overeat. The first step is to stop praising the cleaned plate.

- If your child regularly leaves a lot of uneaten food, it may help to put smaller portions on his or her plate.
- Let your child know that it is all right to stop eating if he or she feels full. This encourages children to respond to their own hunger and satiety cues.
- Draw your child's notice to how you eat more slowly as you become full. Refuse seconds if you're no longer hungry. And avoid saying: "I'm full, but this is so good that I can't stop eating it."

Remember that your child is watching what others do and listening to what they say. If parents and siblings all model healthy eating habits, a pre-school child will have lots of good examples to follow.

One-day menu planner **for pre-school children**

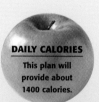

DAILY CALORIES
This plan will provide about 1400 calories.

These sample menus reflect a pre-school child's need to eat frequently throughout the day. Note that the planner includes at least two servings of milk – some with cereal for breakfast, some in the fruit smoothie for the mid-morning snack, and a full serving for the evening snack. If you find your child cannot drink a full serving in one sitting, you can offer milk in smaller amounts during the day.

breakfast
- small glass of fruit juice diluted with water
- fortified cereal with milk
- toast with jam

FOOD GROUP	SERVINGS
carbs	2
dairy	1/2 –1
protein	0
fruits	1
vegetables	0

snack
- 1/2–3/4 serving of strawberry-banana smoothie (see recipe on page 201)

FOOD GROUP	SERVINGS
carbs	0
dairy	1/2 –1
protein	0
fruits	1
vegetables	0

lunch
- baked beans on toast
- a few cherry tomatoes
- small glass of fruit juice diluted with water

FOOD GROUP	SERVINGS
carbs	1
dairy	0
protein	1
fruits	0
vegetables	1

snack
- banana sandwich (1 small banana and 1 slice of bread)

FOOD GROUP	SERVINGS
carbs	1
dairy	0
protein	0
fruits	1
vegetables	0

tea
- pasta shapes with meat sauce (see recipe on page 199)
- green beans
- cubes of melon

FOOD GROUP	SERVINGS
carbs	2
dairy	0
protein	1
fruits	1
vegetables	1

snack
- 175ml (6floz) milk

FOOD GROUP	SERVINGS
carbs	0
dairy	1
protein	0
fruits	0
vegetables	0

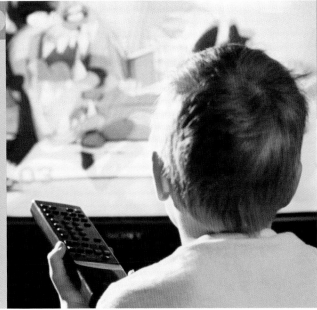

Children hear the fast-food message

A comprehensive review of research into food promotion and children, published in 2003 by the Food Standards Agency, concluded that advertising does affect children's food choices and behaviour, and not just which brands but the types of food they choose. Several studies have found a clear link between the amount of television watched and diet, obesity, and cholesterol levels. So there are good reasons to limit your child's TV-watching. Here are some guidelines:

- Allow your child to watch television for no more than two hours a day.
- Choose non-commercial TV or videos to limit exposure to advertising.
- Look for opportunities to teach your child about TV and other advertising and how it can make some products, including food and drinks, seem more exciting and better for you than they really are.

Letting children have some control

Parents may feel uneasy about giving pre-school kids control over how much they eat. But it's a limited kind of control. The parent is responsible for setting the schedule for meals and snacks and deciding which foods to serve. A child of four shouldn't be getting his or her own snacks, but can be given a choice and allowed to decide whether to eat or not.

There's nothing wrong with serving foods you know your child likes, but they shouldn't always be on the menu. Serve a variety of foods and don't cater to a child's limited palate. It may seem illogical, but it's better to present a range of foods, even if your child sometimes refuses to eat anything on the plate. It's normal to want your child to eat his or her tea, but it's also important to know that skipping one meal will not harm a healthy child. Let the child know food will be available at the next regular meal or snack time – and not before then.

If your child chooses not to eat a meal, try to avoid arguing about it or criticizing the child. Staying neutral and calm will help prevent the more vexing problems that can arise when parents and children battle over eating habits.

Pre-school children who "eat all day"

The average pre-school child eats three meals a day plus two or three snacks. But given the opportunity, many would choose to snack all day long. A child who "grazes" like this might never feel hungry. You want your child to know when

he or she is hungry – and full – because then the child will be better able to regulate how much food to eat. Here are some additional reasons to discourage grazing:

- A child who's hungry at mealtime may be more inclined to try new foods and eat the healthy foods presented.
- Children who graze are often snacking on higher calorie foods and drinks, which put them at risk of excessive weight gain.
- A child who snacks frequently, especially on sweets, is more likely to get dental caries.

Pre-school kids can be easily distracted, so make sure they sit at the table for meals and snacks. Also turn off the TV. And notice if there might be a reason – other than feeling full – why your child is always ready to leave the table quickly. Maybe he or she is in a hurry to get back to playing or leaves the table when an older sibling has finished eating.

Set times for eating are also beneficial because children like having a daily routine. Then they know what to expect. For example, if they start to feel hungry at pre-school, they'll remember that they always get a snack right after story time. Or if they don't feel hungry when it's time for an afternoon snack at home, they'll know that their tea is just around the corner. On a very active day, though, it's perfectly normal for a child to be extra hungry and need more than the usual amount to eat. On those days be flexible if your child wants an extra snack or eats more at mealtime.

When pre-school kids are thirsty

Sugary drinks, such as fizzy colas and squashes, offer very few nutrients but do contain a lot of sugar, which can damage teeth. Even diet drinks can be damaging to teeth. In addition, children who have a lot of sugary drinks are more likely to be overweight and to put on weight because it's easy to drink too much cola and squash. Children are more likely to drink increasing amounts as they get older. Colas also often contain caffeine, which can have negative effects on children (see below).

Pre-school children should not drink sugary fizzy drinks because they can get in the way of good nutrition: they are very filling, so they could reduce your child's appetite for healthy foods that contain the nutrients he or she needs. The best strategy for parents is not to serve colas and other fizzy drinks at all.

Although pure fruit juice offers vitamins that are good for children's health, it also contains a kind of sugar and acid that can damage a child's teeth, which is why it is best to serve juice (diluted with water) only at mealtimes. The best drinks for pre-school children – and indeed for all kids – to have between meals are milk and water. These don't contain added sugar, and milk offers important vitamins and minerals such as calcium. Give whole or semi-skimmed milk until your child is five years old, after which you can switch to skimmed milk if you prefer.

If your child doesn't like plain milk, try making your own milkshakes or smoothies by blending soft fruit, such as banana, strawberries, or mango, with milk or yogurt. This can also be a good way to encourage children to eat fruit.

Decaf kids

Most parents wouldn't dream of giving a pre-school child a cup of coffee, but they may routinely serve cola and other fizzy drinks that contain caffeine. For children, the effects of too much caffeine are similar to those seen in adults:

● jitteriness and nervousness
● upset tummy
● headaches
● difficulty concentrating
● difficulty sleeping.

Because pre-school kids are not very big, it doesn't take a lot of caffeine to produce the effects. Caffeine also acts as a diuretic (something that makes a person urinate more). For young children, especially on hot days, this can contribute to dehydration. (See page 67 for more about dehydration.)

Drink calories **count**

All drinks are not created equal. Milk has more calories than cola, but it's rich in nutrients where cola provides only empty calories. Unsweetened orange juice contains about as many grams of sugars as a juice drink, but the fruit juice is the better choice because it is naturally rich in vitamin C and provides fibre. Choose milk and water most often as between-meal drinks for your pre-school child and limit juice to no more than 150ml (5floz) a day.

DRINK	SIZE	CALORIES	SUGARS
Water	150ml (5floz)	0	0g
Semi-skimmed milk	150ml (5floz)	80	7.5g
Unsweetened orange juice	150ml (5floz)	55	13g
Juice drink	150ml (5floz)	58	15g
Milkshake (from powdered mix)	150ml (5floz)	130	16g
Cola or other sweetened fizzy drink	150ml (5floz)	58	16g

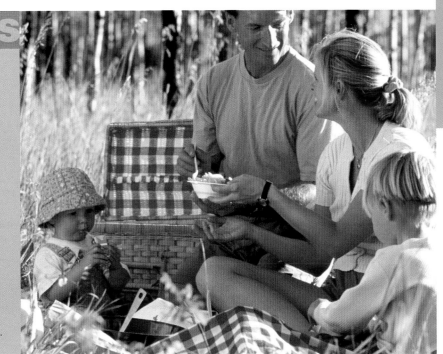

tips

Pack a picnic

A picnic can be a fun adventure for kids of this age. Consider heading to a nearby park or somewhere with a water view. If you can't or don't want to go far, the back garden will do just as well.

- Work together to prepare a list of picnic foods. Be sure to take along at least one fruit and one vegetable per person.
- Let your child help prepare the lunch or pack the cooler. Pack paper plates with characters on them, special cups, or even some silly coloured straws.
- Don't leave home without lots of napkins, hats, sun cream, insect spray, and a big, soft blanket to spread on the ground.

To avoid giving your child too much caffeine, be aware that it is found in other foods. In addition to colas and many other fizzy drinks, caffeine is found in chocolate, coffee ice cream, cocoa, and tea.

Although the UK has not yet developed guidelines for caffeine consumption in children, Canadian guidelines recommend that pre-school children consume no more than 45mg of caffeine a day. This is equivalent to the average amount of caffeine found in a 360-ml (12-floz) can of cola or four 45-g (1.5-oz) milk chocolate bars.

Helping in the kitchen

Involving children in food preparation is a great way to keep mealtimes upbeat and positive. At this age your child's natural curiosity extends to food and cooking, and you can assign him or her small tasks, such as putting ingredients into the mixing bowl or adding the toppings to a quesadilla (see page 193 for a recipe). Unfortunately, though, their curiosity can get pre-school children into trouble in the kitchen, so be sure to keep a close watch on your child when you cook together. Children need to be taught not to touch whirring electric beaters, hot pans, and cookers. There are some simple steps to take to keep your child safe.

- Give frequent reminders about what is okay to touch and which items can hurt them.
- Talk about which kitchen tasks are for grown-ups and which are for kids.
- Establish kitchen rules, such as not touching cooker knobs or picking up knives.

Even as a child gets older, he or she may need reminding about how to work safely in the kitchen. (For more information on this topic, see page 49.)

Having your child help you in the kitchen is a wonderful opportunity for fun and learning. Following a recipe together is a chance for your child to apply maths skills as he or she counts out spoonfuls of nuts and is introduced to fractions. Your child also will enjoy the process of packing a picnic basket (see above for some tips).

It's also a great time in childhood for toys related to food and cooking. Child-size kitchen sets and pretend food items are good choices. Point out the healthy foods in your child's mini kitchen and have your child "prepare" a meal for you. If your child likes to draw, have him or her create a menu card for that night's dinner. You might even have your child take your order and then serve you as if you were in a restaurant. Bon appetit!

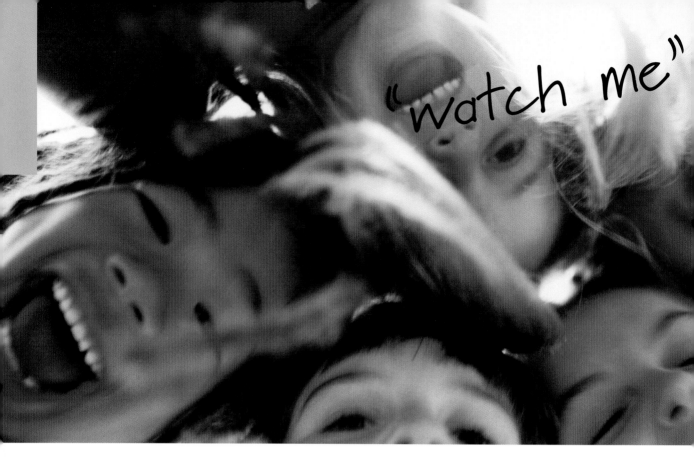
"watch me"

Activity for pre-school kids

Like toddlers, pre-school kids have a lot of energy, but they are able to use it in a more organized fashion. Instead of just running round in the garden they will ride a trike or chase a butterfly.

Pre-school kids need to play

Children of this age are movers and shakers, quite literally. Talk about an airplane and a pre-school child just might thrust out his or her arms and start jetting around the room. Put on some music and your child will be happy to dance.

Pre-school children are also discovering what it means to play with a friend instead of just alongside one, as toddlers do. If your child has spent most of his or her time with family, or the only group experience has been a music and movement class, it's time for your child to branch out and meet new friends. Having this opportunity to be around other children will help your child learn important social skills such as sharing and taking turns. No doubt there will be

disputes, but pre-school children are at an age when they can learn to cooperate and interact while they play. They might play a simple board game, work together on a castle in the sandpit, or play house.

How much activity is enough?

Pre-school children should have at least 30–60 minutes of structured play time every day. In addition, they should get at least one hour – and up to several hours – of free play. They are likely to get structured play at a nursery or their pre-school. They might play "Pass the Parcel" and "Simon Says" or simply practise catching or kicking a ball. They also love a trip to the playground. Just be sure that the equipment is safe and that you keep a close watch on them. (See more safety tips on page 121.) Lots of fun things can be organized indoors, such as setting up a child-friendly obstacle course (see below for this and other activity ideas). Designate a play area and clear the space of any breakables. Or go outdoors and plant a section of the garden together (see page 111).

Unstructured or free play is when the child is left more to his or her own devices – within a safe environment of course. During these times a child should be able to choose from a variety of activities, such as exploring, playing with toys, painting and drawing, doing a puzzle, or dressing-up.

During pretend play, pre-school children often like to take on a gender-specific role because they are beginning to identify with members of the same sex. A girl might pretend to be her mother by "working" in the garden, while a boy might mimic his dad by pretending to cut the grass. It's clear your child is keeping an eye on how you spend your time, so set a good example by exercising regularly. Your child will pick up on this as something parents do, so naturally he or she will want to do it as well.

Helping your child learn new skills

Pre-school children are developing important motor skills as they grow. Some of the new skills your child may be showing off include hopping, jumping forwards (long jump), catching a ball, doing a somersault, skipping, and balancing on one foot for five seconds or longer.

Parents can help their children practise these new skills through playing and exercising together. Here are some ideas for parent-led activities.

- Play follow the leader. Take turns being the leader and mix it up with jumping, hopping, and walking backwards.
- Kick a ball back and forth with your child, or set up a "goal" for your child to aim for.
- Play bounce catch.
- Use paper airplanes to practise throwing.
- Balance a beanbag while walking. Make this more challenging by setting up a simple slalom course.
- Practise balance by pretending to be statues.
- Play musical statues or freeze dance.
- Play wheelbarrow by holding your child's legs while he or she "walks" forward on the hands.

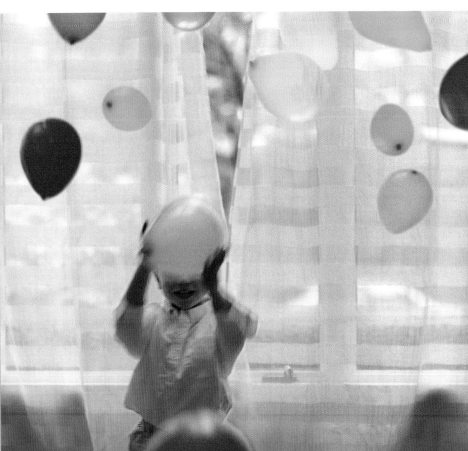

How to keep children active indoors

When children are stuck inside, it's easy for them to get into the TV habit. Instead, try these ideas for keeping them busy.

Treasure hunt Hide little "treasures" throughout your house and give clues where they may be found.

Obstacle course Set up chairs, boxes, and toys for the children to go over, under, through, and around.

Soft toys Use soft foam balls to play indoor netball, ten-pin bowling, football, or catch. You also can play volleyball using a balloon, or play catch with lots of balloons.

Forts and tents Set up a small tent or build a fort out of sheets and cardboard boxes or chairs.

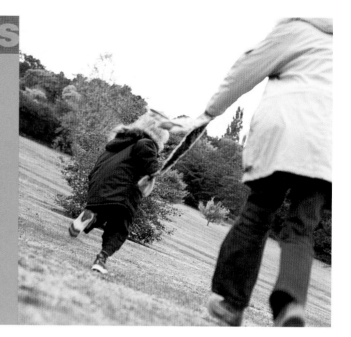

Keep them moving

You know your child has energy to spare, yet when you go out for a family walk, he or she almost instantly complains: "I'm tired!" It's unlikely the child is worn out; he or she is just bored. A brisk walk, while invigorating to an adult, may be dull to a young child. When you're going out the door tell your child you're going on an adventure, treasure hunt, or parade. Then make it fun by using these tactics to liven up your family stroll.

- Set goals such as walking to a nearby park, canal or lake, or friend's house.
- Walk backwards, skip, or jump part of the way.
- Race your child to the next tree or lamp-post.
- Point out interesting bugs, plants, rocks, or clouds.
- Play "I spy" along the way.
- Sing songs or recite nursery rhymes while you walk to your destination.

The very active pre-school child

Some parents worry that their active pre-school child may be hyperactive or have attention deficit hyperactivity disorder (for information about ADHD, see page 179). In fact, these disorders usually aren't diagnosed in pre-school children because it's normal for them to be active and have short attention spans. As children get older, more is expected of them, and it is then that it may become clear that a child is less focused, has poorer judgement, and is much more active than his classmates.

To gauge whether overactivity might be a problem for your child, consider these questions:

- Is your child's activity level unusual for children of the same age?
- Is your child highly active in all settings (home, at pre-school, etc) or just in some settings, such as in church?
- Is your child highly active all or most of the time? Or is it mostly on days when he or she can't go outside to run and play?

If your child is very active, try to avoid situations where he or she is forced to sit still for long periods of time. Also look for safe ways for the child to be active, even if you can't get outdoors (for some ideas about how to keep children active indoors, see page 119). Many pre-school kids will become more calm and focused by the time they reach the early school years. But if you're still concerned about your child, make an appointment with your GP to talk about it.

Getting ready for school

Being active together can be great fun because pre-school children like to learn as they go. A walk outside can become a nature hike as kids notice the leaf floating in a puddle, the beetle crawling across the pavement, and the bird perched on the fencepost. The same walk can become a scavenger hunt if you give your child a list of things to find: a red door, a cat, a flag, and something square. Your walk together can even become a mathematical experience if you emphasize numbers and counting: How many windows are on that house? Do you see any number threes?

Without realizing it, these kinds of activities prepare children to start school. They begin to understand more about the world and how it works. And they can learn basic concepts, such as counting, letters, and colours. Other organized activities such as swimming or dance classes also can help prepare children for the world of school. Through such classes a child can be part of a group and learn to follow instructions, as well as getting a little practice separating from mum and dad for a short while – all important skills to learn for school readiness.

Old enough for team sports?

Many parents are eager to start their pre-school child in organized sports. Although some clubs may be open to children as young as four, organized and team sports are not recommended until a child is a little older. Pre-school children can't understand complex rules and often lack the attention span, skills, and coordination needed.

Instead of learning to play a sport, children of this age should continue to work on fundamental skills, such as hopping on one foot, catching a ball, doing a somersault, and maybe riding a bicycle. If you want to teach your child to play rounders, start by teaching him or her basic skills such as throwing and catching a soft ball. Then, if you play a game, don't expect your child to understand all of the rules or even to follow them. Don't worry if your child doesn't throw the ball to you at the right time – it's enough that he or she is throwing it in the right direction!

Safety concerns

No matter what type of physical activity your child gets, safety remains a concern because pre-school kids are still developing coordination, balance, and judgement. As a parent, you must strike a balance between letting your child try new things while doing what is necessary to keep him or her safe and to prevent injuries.
- A child on a trike or bike should always wear a helmet.
- If you haven't done so already, it's time to talk about road safety because even the most cautious pre-school child may dart into the street after a ball.

- A pre-school child in the swimming pool needs constant adult supervision, even if he or she has learned to swim. It's a tricky age because kids want more independence, and should have some, but they cannot be left unsupervised.

Children this age still need their parents to set limits. For instance, a pre-school child won't know when it's time to take a break on a hot summer day. Likewise, he or she may not know when they have had enough TV or computer time. Pre-school children shouldn't be inactive for more than an hour at a time unless they're sleeping, so it's easy to understand why a lot of TV isn't advisable. It can start a pattern of inactivity that could lead to weight problems or lack of physical fitness for your child.

Should pre-school kids use a computer?

Like watching TV, using a computer is a sedentary activity that should be limited. If your child plays on the computer, make sure the combined TV and computer time doesn't exceed two hours a day. If you decide to allow your child to use the computer, carefully choose the software and the websites your child can visit. Place the computer in a part of the house where you can easily monitor your child and be aware of how long the computer is in use.

Even though many websites and computer games are marketed at this age group, using the computer is not as valuable as other pastimes, such as playing, going outside, talking to a parent, or drawing a picture. As one paediatrician put it: "A computer can't teach values, relationships, self-assurance, or the ability to set goals and to dream."

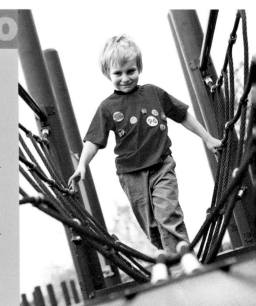

Playground safety

The playground can be a great place for young children to explore and get some exercise. To keep your child safe, follow these tips:
- Select playgrounds that appear to be in good condition and have soft surfaces for landing (sand, a deep layer of wood chips, or rubber mats).
- Teach your child simple safety rules, such as holding on when using a swing and going feet-first, not head-first, down a slide.

- Supervise your child at all times. Be nearby to help out as your child climbs and uses other equipment that could cause injuries. Children of pre-school age should not climb higher than 1.5m (5ft). Be sure your child doesn't wander outside the play area.
- Direct your child to equipment that is appropriate for his or her age.
- Watch out for open "S" hooks or protruding screws that might snag your child's skin or clothing.

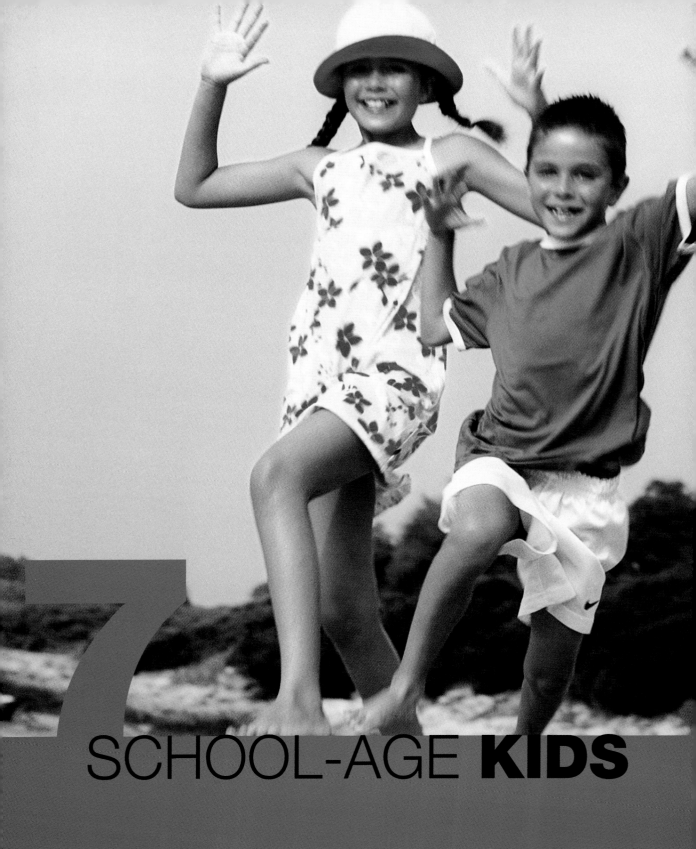

7 SCHOOL-AGE **KIDS**

School-age children are **growing in independence** and are learning to take care of themselves. During these years parents instil **good nutrition and fitness habits** by setting limits and being role models.

age 6–12

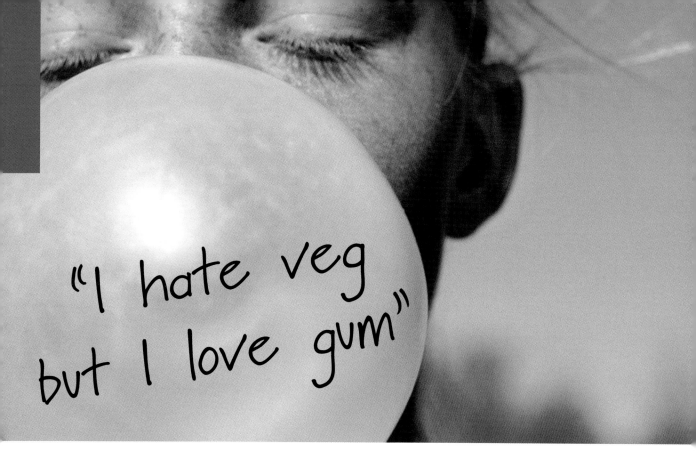
"I hate veg but I love gum"

A time of dramatic change

Between the ages of six and 12, children grow from youngsters still clutching their parent's hand to near-adolescents trying to create their own identities, often in the image of their peers.

Becoming independent

Physical growth continues its steady pace for school-age children, but will pick up dramatically with the onset of puberty, which is usually between eight and 12 for girls and ten to 14 for boys. Good nutrition and adequate physical activity are essential during these years. As children begin to gain more control over what they eat and how active they are, there will be new challenges for parents.

Keep them eating healthily

Although children at this age are making more of their own choices, parents still need to take the lead when it comes to eating so they can steer kids in the right direction. This means providing a variety of nutritious foods for them to choose from, because much of what children eat at this age is still, to a large extent, determined by what is served and stocked at home.

At school, the cinema, birthday parties, and other special events, children may well be influenced by what their friends are eating. It's fine for children to enjoy less nutritious foods from time to time, but the trick is to keep the occasional from becoming the norm. An otherwise healthy diet can help offset the effects of occasional lapses; however, this approach doesn't work the other way around. Eating healthy foods once in a while cannot compensate for a diet that lacks balance and proper nutrition.

A positive attitude towards fitness

School-age children need regular physical activity, not just an occasional afternoon of cycling. Parents often look to organized sports to fill this need during the school-age years. These early experiences can cultivate a child's love for a sport like football – or they can create feelings of frustration and inadequacy that lead to a more sedentary lifestyle. It's fine if your child doesn't like team sports or show interest in them. There are plenty of other ways to be active without being a member of a team or club.

Individual activities, such as swimming or walking, may lead to an exercise habit that lasts a lifetime. Skipping or playing tag can provide as much – or more – sustained, vigorous physical activity as a football match. Even if your children are involved in organized sports, make sure they still have time for the fun and frolic of free play. You might even join them once in a while. It's a good chance to teach your children to love physical activity, in whatever form suits them, and they will see it as a pleasure and not a task.

Reassurance helps

Being active improves coordination and strength, helping children develop confidence and a positive attitude about their bodies – feelings that lead to good self-esteem. This is of particular importance for school-age kids, who begin to pay close attention to their bodies and worry about whether they are normal. If they think they are less coordinated, less athletic, or a different size from their peers, this can make them feel out of place. And as they get closer to puberty, children will scrutinize their bodies even more. Some boys may worry that they are smaller and less muscular than their friends. A girl, on the other hand, may fret about her weight or when her period is going to start.

A visit to your GP can provide reassurance for you and your child. A child who is overweight may welcome a chance to talk with the doctor, especially if the child is worried about his or her weight. Dealing with this now also may spare children from being teased and feeling left out, which can be intense for children of school age, especially as they approach adolescence.

If you look around at your child's school, you will see children of various body types and athletic ability. It is important to remember that regardless of their physical characteristics and athletic talents, all children need frequent reminders that they are loved.

Fit for a life change
School-age children need to eat a nutritious and balanced diet and get plenty of regular physical activity to be in the best shape for the great change they face – the onset of puberty.

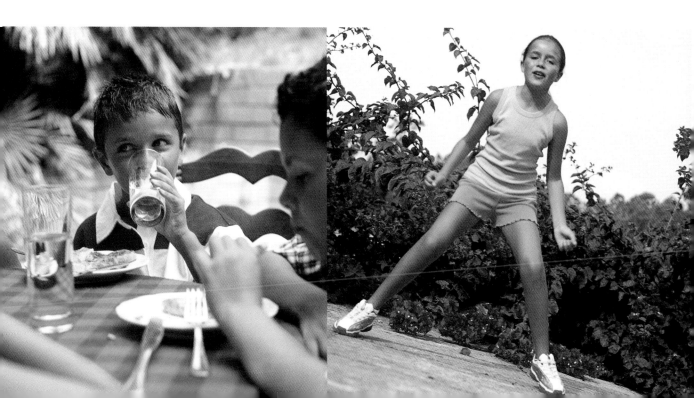

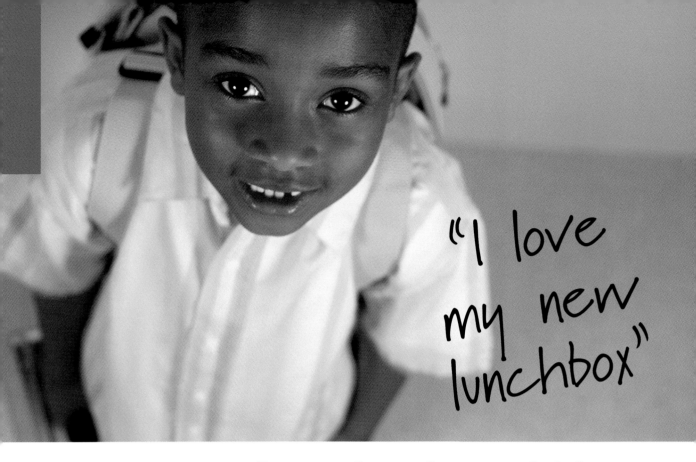

"I love my new lunchbox"

Nutrition for school-age kids

When children start going to school it's an opportune time to give them more control – within parental boundaries – over which foods they eat. Lunchtime and after-school snacks are the places to start.

Making good decisions

Letting children decide what to eat may mean giving them a more active role in food preparation and, as they get older, teaching them to be informed consumers who read food labels and make healthy decisions based on that information (for more about this, see page 48). Help your child make the right decisions now so they can avoid nutrition problems.

- A child who eats too little or doesn't get enough healthy foods is at risk of a nutritional deficiency. Calcium is a concern, especially for children aged nine and older.
- A child who overeats could end up with a weight problem, joining the 30 percent of children already struggling with too many pounds.

Nowhere is decision-making more challenging for children than in the school dining hall. Prepared school meals may offer balance and portion control when eaten in their intended form, but children often have other options that allow them to overeat or eat too much of one food. Fast foods, sweets, and fizzy drinks are readily available at or near schools and are difficult for many young people to resist. Packing a child's lunch or helping him or her pack a healthy lunch, and a healthy snack for after school, enables you to stay in the driving seat when it comes to lunchtime and after-school nutrition. After-school snack attacks can be another problem, particularly for older kids who may come home before their parents do (see page 134).

Daily nutrition needs

Here are the dietary requirements for school-age children. You'll notice that as they get older they will eat more and take in more calories, so the total amount of each component increases. A child who's very active, tall for his or her age, or participating in competitive sports may need more calories than the recommended amount. Use these figures as a guide as opposed to tracking them gram by gram. (See the sample daily menu planners on pages 130 and 133 for ideas on how to put the requirements for your child's age group into practice.) Remember that nutrition is an average.

DIETARY COMPONENT	CHILDREN 6–8	CHILDREN 9–12
Carbohydrates	200–250g	300g
Protein	20–28g	28–42g
Fat	48–60g	60–75g
Fibre	10–12g	14–17g
Total daily calories	1600–2000 calories	1800–2200 calories

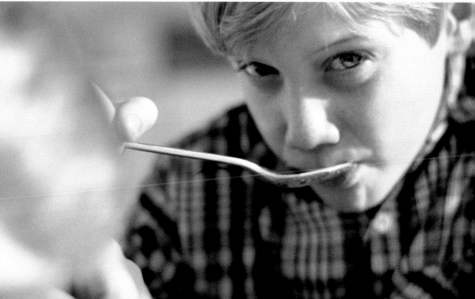

info

Cereal is g-r-r-reat

School-age children will usually get all the vitamins and minerals they need by eating a varied diet. A good way to be sure your child meets his or her daily requirements is by serving them fortified breakfast cereals. Of course, cereal is great for breakfast, but it's also good for quick snacks, especially if the cereal contains little added sugar. And semi-skimmed milk poured on top adds calcium and vitamins A and D, which kids need.

School meals

It's tempting to let your children buy lunch at school each day, but the cafeteria system offered by many secondary schools may allow them to choose a meal that isn't very nutritionally balanced. A packed lunch is often a better choice.

Eating well at school

Statutory nutritional standards for school meals were reinstated in 2001. But while schools in the UK may be required to ensure that the lunchtime meals they provide for their pupils meet healthy standards, most children have the option of mixing choices – choices that tend to be heavy on fat and light on fruit, vegetables, and whole grains. A glance at your child's school dinner menu may show you chicken nuggets, burgers, chips, and sausages on offer.

Schools have taken steps to provide tempting salads and other more nutritious fare, such as grilled chicken, lean beef dishes, and a non-fried carbohydrate option such as baked potato. But even if the prepared meal is a healthy one, it is very easy for children choosing their lunch to bypass the healthy option in favour of pizza, sugary drinks, crisps, and chips. The fact is that while most schools experience few problems in making nutritious food available, it is far harder to persuade pupils to eat it.

Once children reach secondary school they also have access to vending machines whose proceeds buy books or new sports equipment for the school. There are moves now to require that the vending machines be stocked with healthier snacks, but less nutritious options will still be available.

Talk to your child about what lunchtime is like.

- What do they usually eat?
- Are they encouraged to have the full set meal or can they pick and choose freely?
- Is the time relaxed or is it rushed, especially for children who choose to buy a prepared meal?
- Is the dining hall pleasant or is it noisy and chaotic?
- Do children swap foods?
- Do children comment on each other's food, particularly on items in packed lunches?

If you want to improve school meals, a good idea is to talk with other parents and to lobby the school governing body or local education authority for further changes that promote

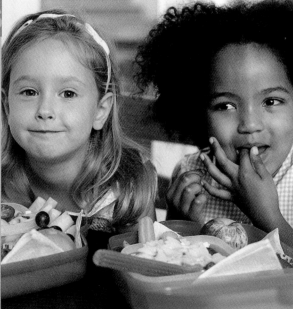

tips

Be on the safe side

It's important to take a few food safety precautions when packing your child's lunches.

- Use a thermos flask for hot foods.
- Use a cold pack to keep cold foods cold. One study found fewer than a third of parents included a cold pack when packing yogurt, meat or fish sandwiches, and other foods that need refrigeration.
- As an alternative to cold packs, you might experiment with freezing some foods and drinks overnight and letting them thaw in the lunchbox.
- Wash out lunchboxes every day or use paper lunch bags that can be discarded.
- Whoever packs the lunch should wash their hands before packing it. Then toss in some moist hand wipes to remind children to wash their hands before eating – and to clean themselves up afterwards.

Lunches at home, at school, and on the go

A lunch eaten at home or brought from home is often the best choice because parents can control the contents by keeping healthy foods to hand or including them in the lunchbox. Here's how a home-made lunch stacks up against a school meal and a typical fast-food meal, in terms of approximate calories and fat content and food group servings provided.

home-made lunch

- turkey on wholemeal bread with lettuce, tomato, and mustard
- 1 banana
- low-fat cereal bar
- 200ml (7floz) semi-skimmed milk

FOOD GROUP	SERVINGS
carbs	2
dairy	1
protein	1
fruits	1
vegetables	1/2

This meal provides 500 calories, of which 23 percent comes from fat.

school meal

- beef and vegetable stew
- bread roll
- apple
- brownie
- 200ml (7floz) semi-skimmed milk

FOOD GROUP	SERVINGS
carbs	1
dairy	1
protein	1
fruits	1
vegetables	1

This meal provides 575 calories, of which 35 percent comes from fat.

fast-food lunch

- cheeseburger
- fries
- chocolate shake

FOOD GROUP	SERVINGS
carbs	3
dairy	1
protein	1
fruits	0
vegetables	0

This meal provides 958 calories, of which 33 percent comes from fat.

healthy eating at school. Be sure to discuss these issues with your child. You can explain why it's important to have a variety of foods at lunchtime and help clear any obstacles that prevent him or her from making healthy choices when at school.

Bringing lunch from home

It's worthwhile encouraging children to eat a packed lunch. Older kids can pack their own, or – if they don't like doing it – you can make it for them, with two rules:

- They must work with you on choosing items to pack.
- They must agree to eat the packed lunch.

Get younger children excited about the idea by buying them a special lunchbox. Though they may not be particularly interested in the nutritional advantages of a packed lunch, you may pique their interest by letting them select and pack foods they like to eat. Make a list of healthy foods for your child to choose from, such as cheese, fruit, raisins, and nuts, and let him or her pick which ones to pack. Leftovers from last night's dinner also can be a good choice. When children like what's in their lunchboxes, they'll eat more, giving them

the energy they need to learn and play. If your child has an after-school sports practice, the lunchbox is the perfect place to pack an extra snack and drink.

Healthy packables

Ready-prepared lunches for kids usually include a juice drink and a sweet, making them high in calories. It's easy and often cheaper to create your own versions at home with healthier ingredients. Pack them in plastic containers or resealable plastic bags. Here are some ideas.

- wraps (turkey, ham, or roast beef with lower-fat cheese rolled up in a flour tortilla)
- pizza (mozzarella and pizza sauce on a muffin)
- cracker sandwiches (whole-grain crackers filled with peanut butter or cream cheese)
- peanut butter and celery sticks
- crudités with low-fat dip or dressing
- 100-percent fruit juice box
- optional sweet, such as fruit jelly, fresh fruit, low-fat yogurt, oatmeal raisin cookie, or digestive biscuit.

Helping six- to eight-year-olds eat healthily

During the pre-puberty years, seize the opportunity to affect your child's eating habits and attitude towards food as this will have lifelong benefits. Let your child get involved in shopping and meal preparation, and start teaching him or her about good nutrition.

Leading by example

Children this age need the same variety in their diet as younger ones do, but now they are more able to understand why nutritious food is important to their health and general well-being. You are just the person to guide them in this because at this age children still want to please their parents and often follow their lead. If young school-age kids begin to understand nutrition – even at a very basic level – they will be able to apply that knowledge to the choices they make on their own, such as when they are in the school dining hall. To encourage good decisions, create a healthy eating chart at home so your child can track progress towards the goal of eating five servings of fruits and vegetables every day. You can help your child meet this goal by stocking fruits and vegetables at home. Also, help your child eat a healthy diet by serving a variety of foods that meet his or her nutritional needs. Talk – in terms your child will understand – about why making the right food choices is important.

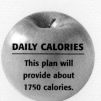

DAILY CALORIES
This plan will provide about 1750 calories.

One-day menu planner **for children six to eight**

No single menu can account for a child's individual tastes and preferences, so don't feel limited by the foods presented below. Use this menu planner to help you get a feel for the amounts and types of food that a young school-age child should be eating. You also can use this format for a food log to analyze your child's diet for a week or so, but don't feel pressure to analyze each day in this detailed way. Instead, keep your eye on the big picture.

breakfast
- 150ml (5floz) apple juice
- 3 tbsp whole-grain low-sugar cereal
- 200ml (7floz) semi-skimmed milk
- 1 slice of wholemeal toast with jam or savoury spread

FOOD GROUP	SERVINGS
carbs	2
dairy	1
protein	0
fruits	1
vegetables	0

snack
- 1 banana or other favourite fruit

FOOD GROUP	SERVINGS
carbs	0
dairy	0
protein	0
fruits	1
vegetables	0

lunch
- tuna sandwich (2 slices of wholemeal bread, tuna, cucumber)
- slices of raw carrot
- 150g (5oz) low-fat yogurt
- 1 tbsp raisins

FOOD GROUP	SERVINGS
carbs	2
dairy	1
protein	1
fruits	1
vegetables	1

snack
- 200ml (7floz) semi-skimmed milk
- 1 slice of wholemeal toast with peanut butter

FOOD GROUP	SERVINGS
carbs	1
dairy	1
protein	0
fruits	0
vegetables	0

supper
- 2–3 fish fingers
- 2 heaped tbsp pasta
- 3 tbsp peas
- a few cherry tomatoes
- small portion of apple crumble with custard

FOOD GROUP	SERVINGS
carbs	1
dairy	0
protein	1
fruits	1
vegetables	2

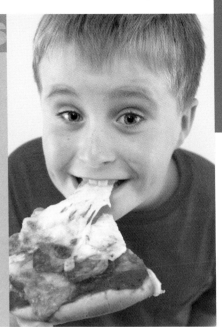

tips

Make your own pizzas

Pizza is popular with children of all ages (adults too) and it's easy to make. Kids will particularly enjoy eating pizza they've made themselves. Here are some ideas for bases and toppings.

- **Bases** (choose wholemeal if possible): prepared thin-crust pizza base, individual-size pizza bases, muffin halves, bagel halves, and pitta bread.
- **Sauces:** pizza sauce (home-made, canned, or bottled), olive oil, pesto sauce, salsa, and barbecue sauce.
- **Toppings** (precook all meats, seafood, and some vegetables, depending on desired crunchiness):

artichoke hearts, green, red and yellow peppers, broccoli, carrots, cauliflower, olives, aubergines, onions, mushrooms, new potatoes, spring onions, spinach, fresh or sun-dried tomatoes, courgettes, sweetcorn, pineapple, shredded chicken and turkey, lean ham, turkey sausage, prawns, canned tuna, and lean minced beef.

- **Cheeses:** mozzarella, mild Cheddar, Parmesan, pecorino, and Gruyére.
- **Seasonings:** pepper, fresh garlic or garlic powder, fresh ginger, oregano, thyme, basil, rosemary, and dried chilli flakes.

Doing it for themselves

Another way to teach children about making good choices about food is to involve them in the process of preparing it, both for themselves and for the family. Cereal may be one of the first "meals" your young child is able to prepare independently, but it can be the first of many.

Invite your child to help you choose recipes for a family supper, select foods at the supermarket, and cook the meal. Your child might even be able to do some of this on his or her own, especially if you choose something easy to start with such as pizzas (see above). A pizza party is a great introduction to what cooking is all about. Add to the fun by inviting a few of your child's friends over.

Create a pizza assembly line in your kitchen. Have the components – bases, sauces, cheeses, toppings, and seasonings – prepared in advance and set them out on the worktop so the children can select their own. The novelty of being able to choose from a variety of ingredients may encourage your child to try foods he or she otherwise wouldn't. As you work, talk about how varied selections can pack the pizza with nutritional punch: for example, a wholemeal base will provide complex carbohydrates; broccoli offers vitamins and fibre; and cheese is rich in calcium. Explain the cooking process – what oven temperature for how long – and let the children decide if the pizza should be soft in texture or crusty. When the pizzas are ready, sit down together, applaud the children for a job well done, and enjoy their efforts. Take time for a little conversation too.

Snacking before mealtimes

Strategic, healthy snacking is better than letting children get too hungry, especially if they must wait several hours before getting their evening meal. The hours after school are often spent doing homework or attending sports practices or after-school clubs. Children need a nutritious snack to keep them from getting tired and grumpy when they need to be focused and alert.

Another advantage of snacking before a late tea is that your child won't come to the table so hungry that he or she overeats. Rather than a snack, if you're serving soup or a salad you might allow your child to eat these early, before the main meal is on the table.

It's good to get your child into the habit of asking permission before diving into snacks, but start letting him or her make the snacks whenever possible. Offer healthy snacks such as fruit, cheese and biscuits, or peanut butter and celery (turn to page 134 for a list of more healthy snack ideas). With a little coaching, children can learn to wash fruits and vegetables, put peanut butter on celery, and open a yogurt without too much trouble (and only a few splatters).

Keeping nine- to twelve-year-olds eating well

Boys and girls at this age are nicknamed "tweens" because they're between stages – not quite children anymore but not yet teenagers. For most children the first signs of puberty will occur during these years, bringing increased appetite and nutritional needs.

Growing up

The growth spurt that marks the passage through puberty starts, on average, at 10½ for girls and 12½ for boys. As growth picks up, calorie needs grow too. This is especially true for boys. Children at this time generally require an additional 200–300 calories per day. If they are very active, they'll need even more calories. Athletic children may require as many as 2500 calories a day or more during these years.

Getting enough calcium

Boys and girls aged seven to ten need 550mg of calcium per day. But around the age of 11, due to the onset of puberty, their needs for this mineral increase, to ensure the development of healthy bones – to 800mg of calcium for girls and 1000mg for boys. Milk is a great source of calcium, but some children this age dislike milk and may refuse to drink it, or they may be unable to drink milk because of lactose intolerance (for more about this, see page 175).

Here are some calcium-rich alternatives to milk:

- 100g (3½oz) canned sardines in tomato sauce (460mg calcium)
- 50g (2oz) Cheddar cheese (360mg calcium)
- 150g (5oz) low-fat yogurt (240mg calcium)
- 200ml (7floz) calcium-fortified juice (144mg calcium)
- 50g (2oz) almonds (120mg calcium)

Raising informed consumers

If your children are interested, show them how to read food labels (see page 48). And send the message that eating the right foods will help a child feel good and grow properly. That message is especially important as they move from primary school to secondary school and start making more of their own choices about what to eat. Peer groups wield more influence and no one likes to be seen as different during these years. As a result, it may be difficult for a child to make healthy choices, in the school dining hall for example.

What parents say...
about food at home

"I try to cook well-rounded meals and we rarely eat fast food (I can't stand it so the kids never got too used to it). I don't keep cola or junk food in the house either, but of course they sometimes have it when we go out or they are out with friends. Nothing is 'off limits'. I just try to teach them to eat some things in moderation. It is also important for us to sit down together for family dinner. So even with a crazy schedule, we manage to eat together most nights, even though it is usually at 8.30 pm.

"Both of my daughters are aware of how important it is to be physically fit but not to go overboard with slimming and such. They know that the models they see are airbrushed pictures and that the really thin images and girls on TV are not necessarily healthy. Fitness has always been part of my daughters' lives."

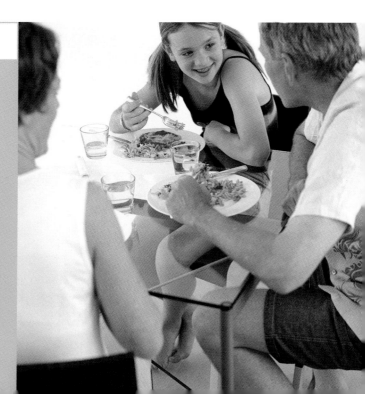

One-day menu planner **for children nine to twelve**

DAILY CALORIES
This plan will provide about 1900 calories.

More than any other age group, this is a time when you may notice a dramatic difference in the amount of food your child eats, even when compared with other children of the same age. The biggest factor will be the onset of puberty, when the older school-age child's appetite will take a sudden upswing. Use the following one-day menu planner as a guideline and adjust it when your child's calorie needs increase.

breakfast
- 150ml (5floz) calcium-fortified orange juice
- 6 tbsp whole-grain low-sugar cereal
- 200ml (7floz) semi-skimmed milk

FOOD GROUP	SERVINGS
carbs	2
dairy	1
protein	0
fruits	1
vegetables	0

snack
- 1 apple or other favourite fruit

FOOD GROUP	SERVINGS
carbs	0
dairy	0
protein	0
fruits	1
vegetables	0

lunch
- ham and cheese sandwich (2 slices of wholemeal bread, cheese spread, wafer-thin ham, sliced tomato)
- red pepper strips
- 250ml (9floz) yogurt drink
- 1 low-fat cereal bar or biscuit
- 1 tangerine

FOOD GROUP	SERVINGS
carbs	3
dairy	1
protein	1
fruits	1
vegetables	1

snack
- 1 small wholemeal pitta bread with reduced-fat hummus
- 200ml (7floz) semi-skimmed milk

FOOD GROUP	SERVINGS
carbs	1
dairy	1
protein	0
fruits	0
vegetables	0

supper
- 50–75g (2–3oz) roast chicken
- 6 tbsp cooked mixed vegetables
- 75g (3oz) mashed potatoes
- small portion of rice pudding

FOOD GROUP	SERVINGS
carbs	2
dairy	0
protein	1
fruits	0
vegetables	2

Peers are not the only ones with the power to influence what your child eats. Advertisers of food and drinks have recognized the buying power of kids. Just watch a little Saturday morning TV. Many adverts tell children they will be cooler, stronger, and more fun if they eat or drink the advertised products. Unfortunately, these sugary drinks, high-fat snacks, and high-calorie foods offer little nutritional value.

Help your child become an informed consumer by questioning the claims adverts make. Also encourage him or her to start comparing labels on advertised foods with other healthier ones. Your child may still want those foods, but you have given him or her a new way of looking at advertising.

Busy schedules
During the later school-age years, children usually have many demands on their time. Football matches or music lessons can interfere with your plans for a healthy supper, but don't give up on eating as a family. Keep beating the drum about shared meals, healthy snacks, and a varied, nutritious diet. Both kids and parents need them even more during these busy years. Stock up on easy snacks that you can toss in your child's backpack. Try muesli bars, fresh or dried fruit, and trail mix (there's a recipe for this on page 200).

Quality time together
Making supper together accomplishes the dual goals of spending quality time with your child and everyone eating a well-balanced meal. Consider planning an ethnic food night at home. It may be more fun if you let your child invite a friend round that night. Spend time together looking for recipes, then make a trip to an ethnic market to get the ingredients you need. If the meal is a hit, consider venturing out to try the same cuisine at a restaurant. And get your child involved in choosing other ethnic themes for future meals.

How to keep snacking under control

As school-age children get older, they grow more independent and capable of taking care of themselves. But left to their own devices they may not always make healthy decisions, especially when it comes to snacks after they get home from school.

The snack attack

After a long day, children need fuel to get them through to their evening meal. After-school snacks can be part of a nutritious diet. The trick is providing the right food in the right amount. A perfect snack will ease after-school hunger pangs, but not so much that the child loses interest in eating supper.

If making their own choices, children – and in particular the latchkey child who lets himself or herself into an empty house after school – may opt for crisps and a fizzy drink in the hours before mealtime. Solve this problem by limiting the kinds of snacks available. Make it easy for your child by keeping fresh fruit and cut-up vegetables in plain sight. Don't keep high-fat, sugary, or salty snacks in the house – or store them in an out-of-the-way spot. You also might try preparing an after-school snack the night before so your child can grab it out of the fridge when he or she arrives home.

If your child seems "starved" after school, look into what he or she is eating – or not eating – for lunch. Your child might be spending dinner money on something other than food, tossing out an undesirable packed lunch, or just not getting enough to eat at mealtime.

Coming home to an empty house also can lead some children to snack too much. They might be bored or may not have the judgement necessary to be without adult supervision. Even a child as old as 11 or 12 may not be ready to be left alone. Look for alternatives, such as after-school clubs or spending time at a neighbour's house. The less time a child spends alone, the less time to snack.

Kids like to snack
Parents need to keep an eye on what children are eating. No food should be forbidden – not even ice cream – but it's not a good snack for every day.

tips

Healthy snacks

Children can easily brand nutritious snacks as yucky if they try a food you call "healthy" and don't like it. To avoid this serve a variety of nutritious snacks and be responsive when your child really likes one of them – or really doesn't. Keep the snack menu fresh by serving new items occasionally. If your child tires of a snack, let him or her help choose new ones. Some great snacks for after-school munchies are:

- low-sugar breakfast cereals
- lower fat, lower sugar cereal bars
- rice cakes and corn cakes
- muffins, bagels, and pitta breads
- home-made American-style fruit and bran muffins
- microwave popcorn
- low-fat tortilla chips

- peanut butter – great spread on apple slices or whole-grain crackers
- raw vegetables (broccoli, celery, carrots, cauliflower, cucumber, green beans, mange-touts, and courgettes) with a yogurt-based dressing or hummus for dipping
- fresh fruit (apples, apricots, bananas, berries, grapes, melon, grapefruit, nectarines, peaches, pears, oranges, and pineapple) with cream cheese or yogurt for dipping
- fruit salad
- dried fruit (apples, apricots, bananas, and raisins)
- hard-boiled eggs
- low-fat cheese
- smoothies made with milk or low-fat yogurt and fruit

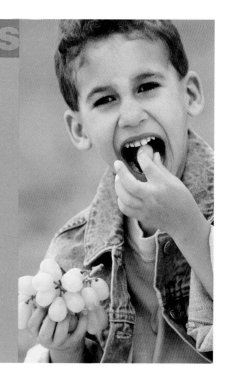

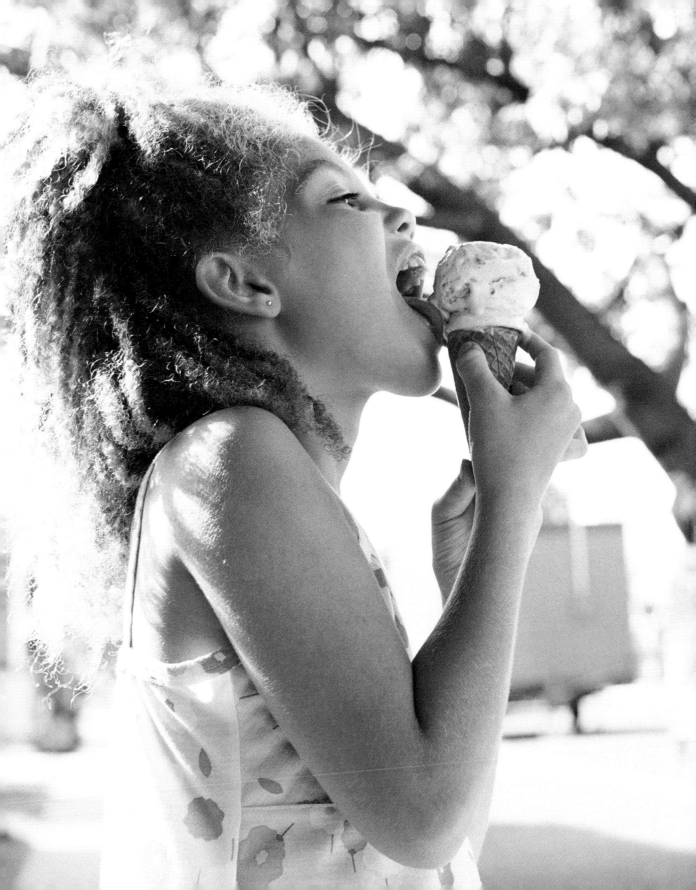

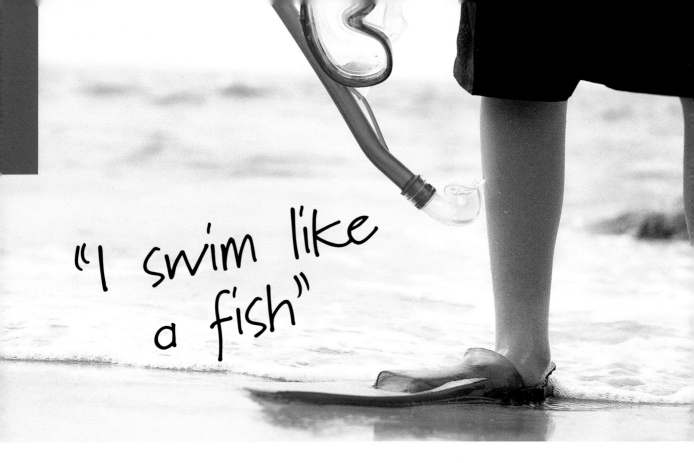

"I swim like a fish"

Fitness for school-age kids

Don't worry if your child doesn't like team sports or show much interest in them. He or she simply may prefer free play to organized games or like individual sports such as swimming and cycling.

The benefits of physical activity

With school-age children spending more time on sedentary pursuits like watching TV and playing computer games, the challenge for parents is to help their children find physical activities they enjoy and feel successful doing.

For some children, their preferred activity may be in a traditional area such as gymnastics or being on the football or netball team. Other children may be fast runners – or they may find they have a great talent for hopping on one foot. Many school-age children enjoy scouting, camping, and other outdoor pursuits, which get them outside and teach them valuable skills. The real challenge comes with those children who dislike all forms of exercise.

Whatever they like to do, school-age children should be active every day. That means at least 30 minutes of physical activity, including ten- to 15-minute bursts of more vigorous activity. This can be time spent in a PE lesson or at break, practising an organized team or individual sport, or playing outside with friends. School-age children also should participate in an additional 60 minutes or more each day of age-appropriate activities, which can include anything they like to do such as putting on a play, playing shopkeepers, looking for bugs, or building a chair tent or a tree house.

Expose your child to a variety of activities, games, and sports so he or she can get the recommended amount of activity every day. School-age children don't care about activity recommendations, but they won't object to being physically active if they're having fun. Make yourself part of the action and keep your child moving by:

- organizing family outings;
- letting him or her take classes to learn different sports;
- taking your child to the playground after school;
- leaving time for free play;
- setting aside some time to be active with your child.

For the child who would rather be reading, listening to music, or playing video or computer games, you might try an incentive chart that offers small rewards such as stickers for every day he or she gets some exercise. (See pages 60 and 138 for more information about how to create an activity log to motivate children.)

In the early school-age years, while children are learning basic skills and simple rules, there may be only a few athletic standouts. As they get older, differences in ability become more apparent. Commitment and interest level often go along with ability, but it's possible for any child to be intensely committed to a sport. It's also possible for a very talented athlete to lack interest. Help your child choose the activity that is right for him or her (see below).

Choosing an activity **that suits your child**

Different sports emphasize some skills over others. The chart below shows a variety of sports and activities alongside the physical and mental abilities needed. You can use this information to find an activity that suits your child's strengths and the areas in which he or she wants to improve. If your child doesn't have much endurance and wants to try the swimming team, what better way to improve stamina than competitive swimming?

SPORT	STRENGTH	FLEXIBILITY	COORDINATION	CONCENTRATION	BODY CONTROL	QUICKNESS	STAMINA
TEAM							
rounders	✓✓	✓	✓✓✓	✓✓	✓	✓✓	✓
rugby	✓✓✓	✓	✓✓	✓✓	✓	✓✓	✓✓✓
basketball	✓✓	✓	✓✓✓	✓✓✓	✓✓✓	✓✓✓	✓✓✓
football	✓	✓	✓✓✓	✓✓✓	✓✓	✓✓✓	✓✓✓
hockey	✓✓✓	✓	✓✓✓	✓✓✓	✓✓✓	✓	✓✓✓
INDIVIDUAL							
swimming	✓✓	✓	✓	✓	✓	✓	✓✓✓
skating	✓	✓✓✓	✓✓✓	✓✓✓	✓✓✓	✓	✓✓
rollerblading	✓	✓✓	✓✓✓	✓✓	✓✓✓	✓	✓✓
dancing	✓	✓✓✓	✓✓✓	✓✓✓	✓✓✓	✓	✓✓
gymnastics	✓✓	✓✓✓	✓✓✓	✓✓✓	✓✓✓	✓	✓
cycling	✓✓	✓	✓✓	✓✓	✓	✓	✓✓✓
running	✓	✓✓	✓	✓✓	✓	✓✓✓	✓✓✓
golf	✓	✓	✓✓✓	✓✓✓	✓✓✓	✓	✓
tennis	✓	✓	✓✓✓	✓✓✓	✓✓✓	✓✓✓	✓✓
fencing	✓	✓✓	✓	✓✓✓	✓✓✓	✓✓	✓
martial arts	✓	✓✓✓	✓	✓✓✓	✓✓✓	✓	✓

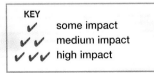

KEY
✓ some impact
✓✓ medium impact
✓✓✓ high impact

Helping six- to eight-year-olds be fit

Parents love to watch their infants and toddlers grow and develop – we know what to expect and can measure the rapid progress. But it's easy to forget that older children pass through developmental stages too.

Encouraging exercise

Between the ages of six and eight, children are learning and mastering fundamental physical skills, such as jumping, throwing, kicking, and catching. It will take a few more years before most children can combine these skills, to throw on the run, for instance, the way many 11-year-olds can. They aren't ready for the pressure of competition and they can't grasp complex strategy.

Now is the time to teach your child basic skills, simple rules, and a sense of accomplishment. Your aim is to create a foundation that will help your child develop a lifelong love of exercise and physical activity.

Free play

When you were a child, you probably did quite a bit of free play, though no one called it that. Free play isn't something a child takes lessons in or needs special equipment for. It's what children do naturally when given the opportunity to decide how to spend their time outdoors. Free play includes hopscotch, skipping rope, dancing, tag, scavenger hunts, and cycling, to name just a few.

Encouraging free play may seem challenging at first, but left to their own devices and creativity it's amazing what children will come up with. And nothing encourages free play like turning off the TV and computer. You can also help by reminding your child that it's time to go outside and by having a selection of games, toys, and sports equipment always on hand (see opposite for some suggestions). In warm weather, sprinklers and hosepipes can inspire a lot of darting and dashing. If the back garden loses its charm, you can simply branch out to nearby playgrounds, parks, and sports grounds. On snowy days, bundle up and head outside to make a snowman or have a friendly snowball fight.

Free play may involve more vigorous activity than PE or a team sport, where a child may spend 20 minutes being active and the rest of the time on the bench, changing into

What parents say...
about motivating kids

"I have two kids, a girl eight and a boy ten, and we were looking for a fun way to get them up and moving. So we decided to make a weekly activity log, to keep track of how active they are each day. We all created the chart together. We put the days of the week across the top of the chart and then listed our kids' favourite activities down the left side (both free activities and more organized sports). Our daughter's choices were swimming, hopscotch, and dancing. Our son opted for riding his bike, playing football, and skateboarding. Every day our son or daughter did one of the activities we put on a star or a sticker. The chart idea was so successful at motivating them we decided to carry on for a month. And we set a goal for each of them to achieve during the month. The reward for reaching their goal was to let them choose a family outing, such as going to the cinema."

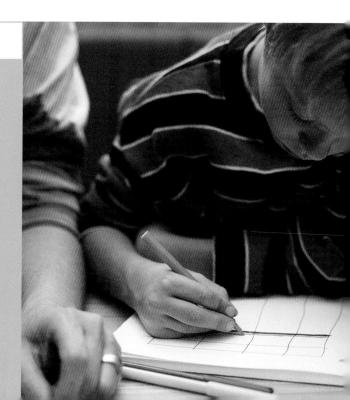

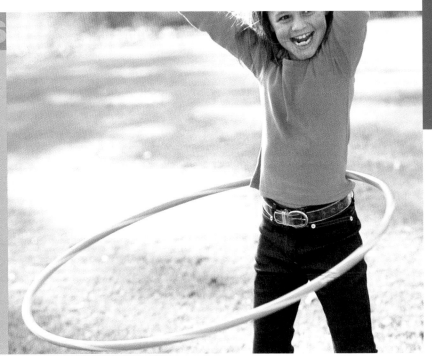

tips

What's in the cupboard?

Having a lot of games and sports equipment on hand encourages children to play. Here are some ideas:
- basket ball or net ball
- rugby ball
- football
- cricket or rounders bat and ball
- pogo stick
- kite
- badminton set
- frisbee
- rubber rings
- pavement chalk
- skipping rope
- hula hoop
- roller skates
- tennis balls and raquets
- croquet set.

his or her kit, or lining up. Studies also show a decline in the frequency of PE classes as well as the amount of physical activity during an average class. It's a good idea to learn more about the physical education programme at your child's school. Here are some steps to take:

- Inquire about how PE lessons are run in your child's school and how active they are.
- Let the school know that physical activity for your child is important to you.
- Ask whether the staff includes dedicated PE teachers and whether other teachers are asked to volunteer to supervise sessions.
- Help your child be prepared for PE lessons with the right clothes and shoes, so this chance to be active during the school day isn't missed.
- Find out if the PE staff also organizes before and after-school sport and games.

For more information about PE classes, see page 141.

Organized sports

Many young school-age children enjoy organized activities, which can be anything from gymnastics (tumbling) and ballet to volleyball. They offer kids lots of opportunities to be active, learn new skills, and feel good about themselves.

Team sports

Playing on a team can teach children about sportsmanship and teamwork while building self-esteem. But there are many ways team sports can go wrong for a young child. It's not enough for coaches to explain the rules of the game or how to do a particular skill. A child must be emotionally or physically able to do it. At this age there are skills some children won't be able to master. That can lead to a sense of failure and frustration, especially if parents or coaches have unrealistic expectations or are harsh in their judgement of the child's performance.

If you think that participation in a team sport is right for your child, look for classes or clubs and coaches that share your philosophy. At this age the emphasis should be on having fun while learning basic skills and being physically active. Remember that success doesn't mean scoring the winning goal. It means that the child who used to run the wrong way on the pitch now runs the right way and takes a shot at kicking the ball in the net. Or even better the child passes it to his teammate who's closer to the goal.

Non-competitive sports clubs are the best choice for the early school-age child. Although some naturally gifted child athletes may take to competitive sports, for most children it's better to avoid teams that put a lot of emphasis

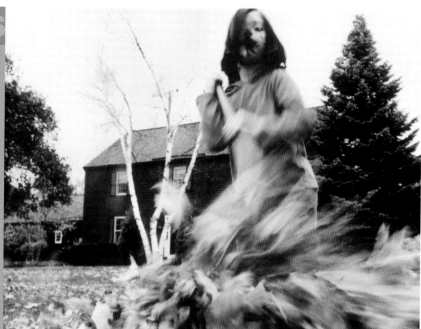

Sneaky exercise

By assigning active household tasks or suggesting outings where exercise just happens, you can sneak physical activity into your child's schedule. Try these:
- cleaning his or her room
- folding laundry
- sweeping or hoovering
- washing the car
- dusting
- watering the garden
- raking up leaves
- shovelling snow off the path or drive
- bird-watching
- shopping
- walking a dog.

on winning. Here are some questions to ask when choosing a sports or activity programme for your child:
- Do all participants get equal playing time?
- Does the coach or leader rotate players so everyone gets a chance to play the more desired positions?
- Does the coach or leader take into account each child's individual needs and abilities?
- Is everyone praised for participating and showing good sportsmanship or are only star players recognized?

Watch for signs your child simply doesn't enjoy practising or playing in the matches. Talk to your child about it and, if necessary, meet with the coach to talk about what it is that's bothering your child.

Team sports have so many potential benefits that many parents are anxious to get their child signed up, dressed in the kit, and on the pitch ready to play. But early failure at any sport may turn children off, causing them to give up on all sport completely because they think they're just not good enough.

Individual sports

Team sports are fine for children who enjoy them, but how many adults regularly play football? Yet long after schooldays are over, many adults continue to enjoy swimming, tennis, running, and cycling – the individual sports and activities they learned in childhood. Like team sports, these promote fitness and give children confidence and control over their bodies. But with individual sports, it's easier for them to set their own pace and improve skills independently.

Of course, the level of intensity will vary from child to child. A child pursuing excellence in gymnastics or skating may have to put in many hours of practice. In fact, these sports depend so much upon repetition that some children do specialize in them, even at a young age. However, a child can get a lot out of gymnastics or skating without trying to pursue an Olympic medal.

Which sport?

To help prevent children from feeling frustrated and giving up, parents can help their child choose the right sport or sports to try. Start by taking into account the child's interests and then consider his or her physical and mental abilities as well as body type. A bigger child might be suited for rugby because size can be an advantage. A smaller child might succeed at cricket or tennis where size isn't such an issue.

Also consider your child's temperament. A mild-mannered boy may not be comfortable playing rugby, but may like the challenge of karate. Likewise, an active girl may not have the patience and control required for ballet, but be better suited to a more fast-paced sport like football.

myth: Physical education (PE) at school provides enough exercise.

fact: Children need regular physical activity to boost alertness at school – an hour a day is recommended – but gym lessons are rarely enough to keep a child fit. At present, only 40 percent of school-age children get two hours of PE a week (adolescents often get even less). In those two hours, time is spent changing clothes, getting instruction, and lining up, all of which reduce the amount of time to be active. During break, there may not be any organized activities to encourage children to move about.

After years of under-investment, many schools have limited sports facilities – or none at all. As a result sporting activities occur away from school, often in hired sports centres, or in exam halls that double as gyms or outdoors in car parks that double as playgrounds. If kids naturally dislike taking part in sport at school because they don't like getting hot and sweaty – or cold and wet – they will be even more unwilling if facilities are poor. If you are dissatisfied with the state of PE at your child's school, try to work with other parents and with teachers and school governors to implement change.

You can guide your children, but remember that the choice of sport should be left largely up to them. As with food, parents can help by presenting the child with a menu of good choices. (See the chart on page 137 for guidelines on how to match your child's abilities with a sport.)

Even if your child is not particularly tall but wants to play basketball, or isn't very strong but wants to do gymnastics, definitely let him or her give it a try. Remember, the goal isn't to produce a star athlete, it's to raise a child who likes being active and is happy to run outside on a sunny day.

Family fitness

Don't just put the onus on your children to be active – make fitness a family affair. If you want your children to keep moving, set the right example by showing them that you enjoy being active as well, especially when it comes to family time. Maybe it's time to take a golf lesson together or make a trip to the tennis court to volley back and forth or spend a rainy Saturday at the local indoor swimming pool. A little friendly family competition can be fun, but don't take it too hard if your ten-year-old beats you!

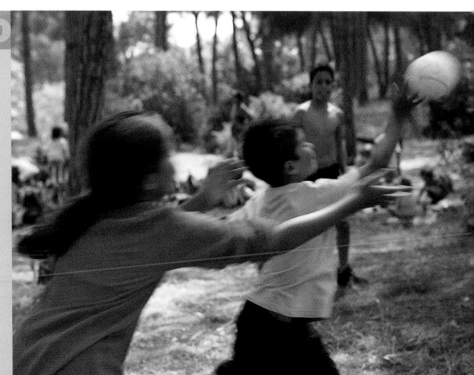

Summer activities and camps

For children, summer is a major change of pace. In one respect, this is good, especially if the school year has been a demanding one. But if summer is too lazy, children may get bored and might not get enough physical activity. One answer is organised activities at your leisure centre or school, or summer camp. There are both residential camps and day camps. They offer a wide range of activities – from all kinds of sport to music and arts and crafts – as well as excursions to places kids enjoy. Whatever kind of activity you choose, your child will have fun being active. When September rolls round, you may find that your child is sad to bid farewell to new friends and can't wait to go back to camp next year.

Keeping nine- to twelve-year-olds physically fit

Being physically active can be exciting for the older school-age child as he or she becomes more coordinated. Whether your child is a natural-born athlete, a casual athlete, or a non-athlete, there are lots of possible sports and activities to try.

Parents can make a difference

All children can refine and improve their skills and feel successful during these later school-age years. Now that they've mastered the fundamentals of their chosen sport or activity, they can work on individual skills, such as improving their back dive, kicking the ball accurately into the corner of the net, or perfecting their free throw. Parents can help at this time by reminding their children that success at sport also includes having fun – and learning how to handle setbacks.

Questions to ask

For children who play team sports, parents need to check that the sports programme is still filling all of the child's needs. There are five important questions for a parent to ask.

- How competitive is this sports club? For nine- and ten-year-olds especially, the right answer is: "We play mainly for fun."
- Is there a policy that every child gets to play at least part of the match? No children should feel left out.
- How often does the team practise? Three nights of practice plus a match each week will be too much for most school-age children.
- How are injuries handled? The coach and assistants should be trained in first-aid and have taken a life-saving course. Referees (umpires) also should be trained in basic safety procedures.
- How can I help? Ask if you can help coach or take on other tasks, such as keeping score, preparing the tea or snacks, and helping with phone calls.

Switching activities

It may have been a few years since you and your child chose a sport or activity from the many available options. The novelty of the new kit may have worn off and it's possible that the activity or sport is no longer the right one for your child. He or she may want to follow their friends into a different activity or just try something new, which is perfectly natural at this age.

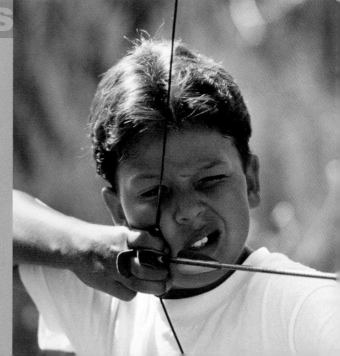

tips

Looking for activities?

Traditional sports and exercise aren't the only way to be active. Here are some alternatives your child might enjoy:
- **Archery** (shooting at a target with a bow and arrow)
- **Baton twirling** (twirling a slim baton, throwing it into the air, and catching it, usually to music)
- **Fencing** (two opponents each use a flexible, narrow, blunt-end sword to attack and defend)
- **Croquet** (players knock wooden balls through hoops on the ground using long-handled mallets)
- **Juggling** (tossing three or more balls into the air and catching them, keeping several in the air at the same time)
- **Golf** (players use long-handled clubs to hit a small ball into a series of holes on a large course)
- **Curling** (teams slide heavy, flat stones along an ice court towards a mark)
- **Indoor rock climbing** (climbing up a sheer imitation rock face with the aid of ropes)

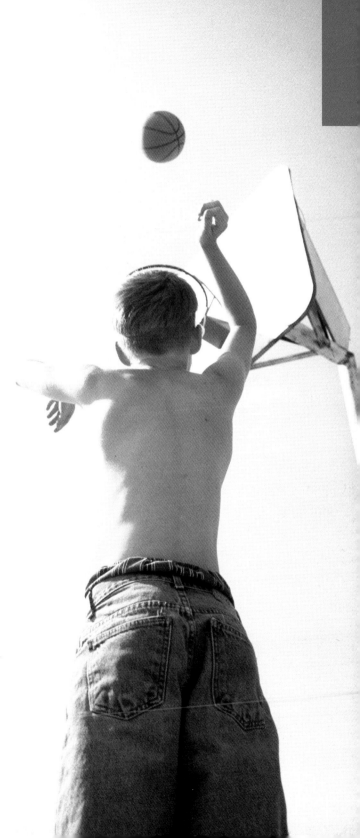

If your child isn't enjoying an activity – or is feeling frustrated by failure – it may be time to switch to something else. That doesn't mean the time spent playing basketball or doing gymnastics was wasted. You should expose your child to a variety of activities and that was just one step along the way. As children grow and change, their activities should reflect what they enjoy and feel competent doing. If they feel sport is a burden, they may choose to be sedentary, putting them at risk of becoming overweight.

Most kids are casual athletes

Some children will want to pursue excellence in a sport, while others may be perfectly happy – and fit – just being casual participants. Most children fall into this latter category, but where there is pressure to be the best it is easy to overlook them as athletes. Yet they stand to gain no matter how well they perform. That's why it's very important to encourage all children to remain active even though they aren't the top performers.

Participation in sport drops sharply between the ages of ten and 18. But why would a child who likes sport lose interest? The answer may be increasing pressure or time requirements (see more about children giving up sport on page 144). If your child is turning away from sport and physical activity, look for ways to make adjustments. Here are some examples:

- A child who loves gymnastics, but doesn't like competitions or the idea of long practices, could be switched to a non-competitive class.
- If a child who loves playing basketball is discouraged because he or she is not scoring as many points as teammates, look for classes he or she could attend and encourage the child to keep practising.
- If a child simply wants to try something new, like rollerblading for example, make sure he or she has the right equipment (see page 65 for information about sports gear), the right instruction, if needed, and a safe place to practise. If the first time out is disappointing – it may well be – encourage him or her to keep trying.

Each child's fitness personality is different
The athlete will want to be on the basketball team, while the casual athlete may just enjoy "shooting hoops" in the playground or on the drive. The non-athlete, on the other hand, is likely to need a parent's help and encouragement to get physically active.

The non-athlete

Some children are not natural athletes and they don't like participating in sport at all. They may shy away from activity because they're overweight and self-conscious about it, or it may be that they aren't as coordinated as their peers. Other children might have a physical condition or health problem that slows them down.

By this age children are aware of these differences and some may have even been teased about them. This may push a child to drop out of a sport or physical activity – something that can hurt his or her confidence. The danger for a child like this is not leaving one activity that didn't work out; it's abandoning physical activity altogether and then becoming a couch-potato kid.

If your child is not interested in physical activity or has given up a sport, try these strategies:

- Look for something new and different to arouse your child's interest (see pages 165 and 203 for some ideas).
- Limit the amount of time used for sedentary pastimes, such as watching television and playing video and computer games. Remember that reading is sedentary too, so suggest your child takes regular breaks from books to move around a bit.

Be helpful and sensitive

Almost all children will be able to find something that they do well enough and feel good about, but the non-athlete may need a parent's help to find that special activity. Start with what you already know your child likes. If the competition of the swimming team proved too much, encourage your child to continue enjoying the sport by swimming at the local pool. Find out which activities his or her friends are doing. Check out what's on offer at the local leisure centre or sports centre and present your child with a menu of possibilities. If possible, make it more appealing by arranging for the child to go to a sports class with a friend. (For more activity ideas, see the list on page 142.)

Cultivate other interests

Every moment of your child's spare time doesn't have to be filled with aerobic exercise. The non-athlete will benefit from having other kinds of scheduled activities that engage his or her interests.

Think about the child's weekly schedule. Can an after-school club fill some unproductive time? For evenings and weekends, you might want to investigate courses at local museums or theatres, as well as music, art, and other

---

info

The child who wants to give up a sport

Giving up can stir emotions for parent and child. If your child is unhappy in an organized sport or activity, the first thing to do is to talk it over with him or her. Remember that it is okay to give up a sport as long as the child gets enough activity otherwise.

In dealing with this dilemma, parents should ask themselves these questions:

- Is my child well suited to this sport?
- Was my child as interested in this sport as I was?
- Does my child have enough unscheduled free time?

Common reasons for quitting include no longer enjoying the sport, feeling too much pressure, or not having enough time for the sport, plus school and other activities. Giving up may be reasonable if the child feels over-scheduled.

After talking with your child, you may find there are steps you can take to improve the situation. You might talk with the coach about problems such as too little playing time. You also might help your child work on improving skills. If he or she wants to keep on with this sport, you might cut another activity out of the schedule to allow some free time during the week. If your child still isn't having fun, it might be time to give up this sport and move on to something new.

Also keep in mind that giving up a sport can be a sign of depression if your child seems sad much of the time and has lost interest in sport and other activities that they usually enjoy. There may be logical reasons why a child no longer enjoys a sport, but if you suspect depression talk with your child's doctor.

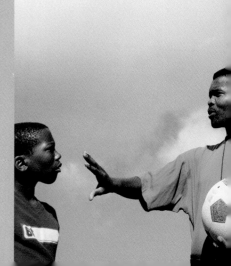

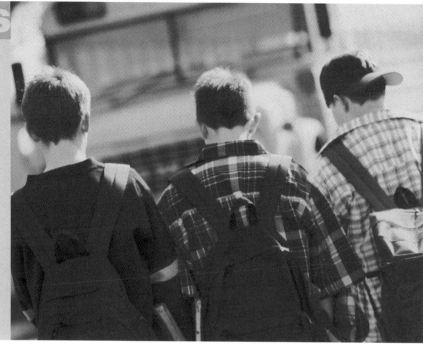

Walking to school

If your child walks to school, ensure the journey is trouble-free. Here are some suggestions for making it safe.

- Teach your child about pedestrian and bike safety.
- Identify the safest route to school.
- Encourage your child to walk or cycle with other children.
- Ask neighbours to keep an eye on children walking to school.
- Make sure your school provides lollipop men or ladies at busy intersections.
- Use the "Walking School Bus" concept, where a designated adult "picks up and drops off" children at their homes (on foot), following a set route.

classes. In summer holidays, keep your child busy at a residential or day camp in your area that will cultivate his or her interests (see page 141 for more about summer camp). Organize family outings and holidays that reflect your child's hobbies. If he likes model trains, go to a local exhibition. If she likes tennis, consider a trip to the lawn tennis museum.

At home continue to encourage "free play" as much as possible by having a variety of sports equipment and games on hand (see page 139 for ideas for what to keep in the cupboard). If your child must be indoors, ping pong, table football, and air hockey aren't going to burn off hundreds of calories, but they're a lot more active than dozing and snacking in front of the television or computer.

The athlete

Some children are happily settled in a sport or activity by the older school-age years. They may have established bonds with coaches, good friendships with teammates, and a solid commitment to their chosen sport. In this situation, a parent can continue to support the child's efforts while watching for any changes. It's important to check that your child:

- is continuing to manage schoolwork;
- is getting enough rest;
- is still enjoying the sport.

Be there if your child wants help practising at home, but think twice before you force it. Practising with a parent can help some children, but others may get fed up if their parents push them too hard. Support your child's club or school team by volunteering to clean up the pitches, make snacks, or participate in fund-raisers. Support your child by attending matches and cheering him or her on from the sidelines, unless they tell you they would feel happier if you weren't there. (Don't take it personally if they say this – many children feel that way.) Avoid making negative remarks about any player or the other team, and never get into squabbles with other parents about whose child is getting more playing time. Leave the coaching to the coach. And don't analyze your child's performance.

Some parents put pressure on their children to specialize in one sport at this age, but this should be avoided at all costs. Instead, let your child try out new things and enjoy a variety of physical activities. Remember that you're trying to develop your child's lifetime love of exercise. It is also important that your child gets some unpressured time, to play other kinds of games and explore other avenues of interest, including those that have nothing to do with sport or exercise. (For more information about the needs of the child athlete, see page 182.)

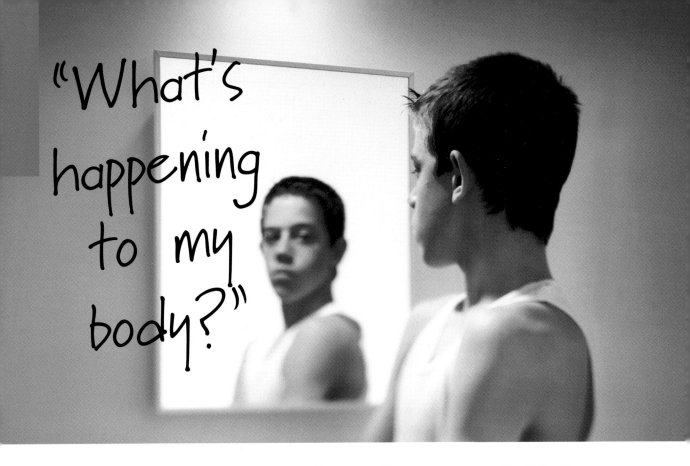

"What's happening to my body?"

Puberty in school-age children

Most children will begin to show the first signs of puberty during these years, at varying times. Early changes can cause fear and embarrassment, which may affect eating and exercise.

Creative parenting required

Growth and development will vary among children, so your ten-year-old may be a lot bigger than his friends. Being bigger can be an advantage in sports such as rugby and basketball, but a disadvantage in gymnastics, which prizes small bodies. The size difference may disappear as other children catch up, and maybe overtake, the early bloomer.

The first changes in puberty, like breast development and pubic hair growth, can make children feel embarrassed about their bodies. They may be reluctant to participate in PE lessons at school because they don't want to change into their sports kit in front of the other pupils. A girl who is developing breasts may be self-conscious and need a bra to make her feel more at ease. Try to keep the lines of communication open, but don't expect children at this age to articulate all their needs. Help them through subtle intervention. Talk to their teachers and coaches too.

While all children go through puberty, their development occurs at such differing rates that it's easy for a child to feel odd because he's the first – or last – to begin developing. Parents need to explain these changes before they happen. Be sure children know that the changes are normal and that it would not be normal for them to get older without the changes taking place. While you're talking about their growing bodies, remind them that good nutrition and physical activity will help them grow up healthy and strong.

Some early signs of puberty

Entering puberty signals the beginning of a host of mental, emotional, and physical changes for a child, but it doesn't happen overnight. In addition to getting taller, here are some of the first changes that occur when a child starts to develop. Boys:

- enlargement of testicles and penis
- hair starts to grow in pubic area
- onset of adult body odour
- skin becomes oilier and acne may begin.

Girls:

- breasts start to bud and grow
- hair starts to grow in pubic area
- onset of adult body odour
- skin becomes oilier and acne may begin.

Gaining weight

It's normal for children to put on some body fat prior to puberty and it's important to reassure any child who thinks he or she is overweight but isn't. However, the child who gains too much now is at risk of being an overweight adolescent. If you think your child might be gaining too much weight, make an appointment with your GP to discuss the issue.

Body Mass Index (BMI) is a helpful tool for monitoring your child's weight. Because it is standardized for height, weight, and age, BMI generally should stay within the normal range while a child is growing. If BMI changes more rapidly than expected, it may be time to take action. Exactly which actions to take will vary from child to child.

Seek your GP's input before putting your child on a diet, which is often inappropriate and unnecessary, and which can be harmful to a growing child. (See pages 18–19 for an explanation of BMI and information about addressing a child's weight problem.)

Watch out for eating disorders

It's normal for children to gain 4.5kg (10lb) or more a year during puberty, but some girls may look at the rising number on the scale and worry they are overweight. They may grow out of their clothes and no longer have the fashionably lean figure seen on magazine covers. A preoccupation with weight and appearance can lead to an eating disorder, such as anorexia nervosa (starving oneself) and bulimia (binge eating followed by self-induced vomiting).

Eating disorders are most common among teenagers, but younger girls who start puberty earlier, especially if they're a little overweight, are at risk as well. The early bloomers are bigger and more mature than their friends, which may make them feel fat. Girls who are uncomfortable with the idea of growing up may fear puberty and view the changes as things they don't want.

Watch for signs that your child is concerned about size and weight, and is taking steps such as slimming or exercising to excess. Note any changes, such as not eating certain foods, skipping meals, refusing to eat with the family, or growing preoccupied with food labels. If you're concerned, discuss it with your GP. You may be able to prevent an eating disorder if behaviours are recognized and addressed early. (For more about eating disorders, see page 163.)

Q: **My daughter is very overweight and wants to attend a weight-loss camp. Should I send her?**

A: It's great that your daughter is motivated to make a change in her life. It could be a positive experience for her to attend a camp where she can meet other children facing the same problem. If your daughter is overweight, she should have already seen the doctor to talk about the best steps to take in attaining a healthier weight. Ask your GP whether this kind of camp might fit into her overall weight-management programme.

Relatively new to the UK, weight-loss camps focus on encouraging healthy eating (not slimming) and on increasing activity levels. Children should learn about proper nutrition and about making better food choices, but they should also focus on having a good time and enjoying the camp experience. Weight-loss camps that take a very rigid approach, where strict discipline about eating and exercise are the rule, should be avoided.

Remember that no camp can completely solve a child's weight problem. When she returns home your daughter will need your help in living a healthier, more active lifestyle.

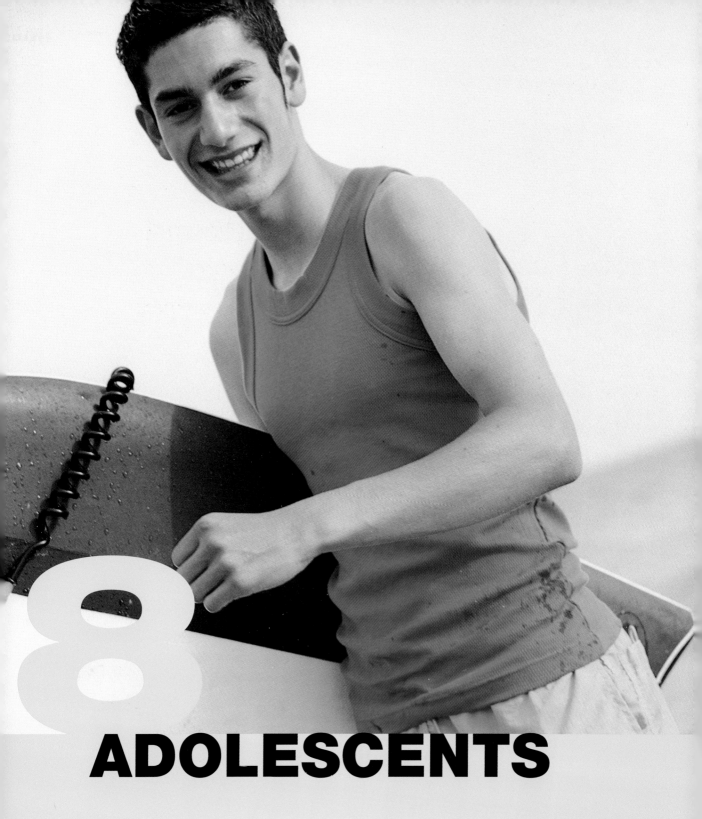

8

ADOLESCENTS

As they **progress towards adulthood** teenagers can learn how to take good **care of themselves**. A teenager's home environment remains an important source of **structure and support** when it comes to **eating and exercise**.

age 13-18

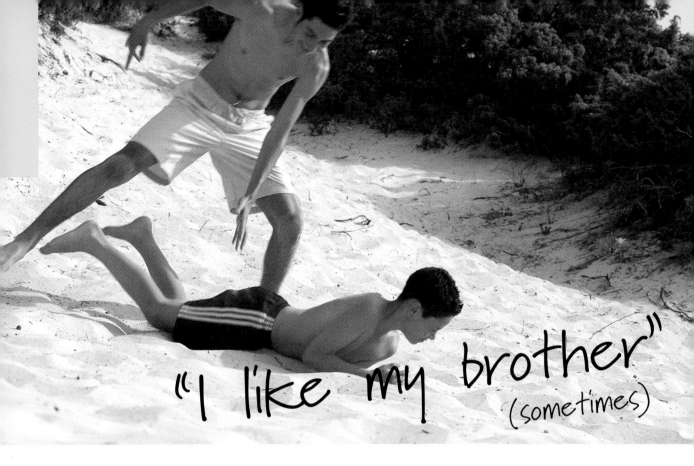

"I like my brother" (sometimes)

Becoming mature

It's true that the teenage years from 13 to 18 are ripe for conflict as it's a time of great change. But these years are also filled with pride and pleasure as you watch your children move towards adulthood.

Teenage challenges

Almost from the moment you bring your new baby home from hospital, you'll start to hear those warnings about the teenage years:

"She's so adorable. Just wait until the boys start ringing."

"Before you know it, he'll be asking for the car keys!"

Once your baby has grown up and is a teenager, you'll understand these comments all too well.

As a normal part of their passage into adulthood, teenagers will align themselves more with their friends and, at the same time, will seem to turn away from their parents. This is a normal stage that allows teenagers to create their own identities. This identity may start out as a carbon copy of their friends, but by the time the teenage years are over, most parents are – more often than not – pleased with the unique finished product.

Rapid growth and big changes

Good nutrition and adequate physical activity are important as children enter adolescence, a period of rapid growth second only to the first year of life. By the start of the teenage years, many girls already have experienced a major growth spurt and have started menstruating (see page 146 for more information about puberty). Most boys, who reach the peak of their growth spurt a year or two later than girls, are in the midst of big changes during these years.

While teenagers' bodies are changing, the way they think about their bodies and themselves is changing too. As they move through the teenage years, they'll begin feeling less self-conscious and more comfortable with how they look. Teenagers are better able to make this transition if they eat healthily and remain physically active.

Your teenager's job is to become an independent person who can make good decisions and take care of himself or herself. You are the guide along the way. If your own approach to eating and exercise is healthy, it will increase the likelihood that your child will adopt and maintain the same good habits for life.

Mum and dad are still role models

Though teenagers say and act otherwise, parents continue to wield strong influence as role models during the adolescent years. One survey found that 65 percent of 15-year-olds said they still wanted their parents' advice and guidance. Parental influence is particularly important when it comes to fitness and nutrition because today an increasing number of teenagers are overweight.

Younger teenagers have a better chance of overcoming weight problems, but older overweight teenagers are more likely to become overweight or obese adults and also suffer the associated health problems (see below and pages 20–23 for information about the medical consequences of being severely overweight). Even if your teenager resists some of your efforts, don't give up on good practices, such as stocking and serving healthy snacks, preparing family meals, and promoting regular exercise habits.

Make every effort to include your teenager in family activities and mealtimes. In addition, always remember that he or she is watching what you do. Your actions and the choices you make may leave a more lasting impression than a lot of long-winded advice or lectures.

It's a fine balance to determine when to give advice and when to let your teenager make the decisions. Adolescence is a time of transition, when a parent needs to relinquish some control, but gradually and within clearly defined limits. A parent needs to remain a constant and consistent presence because even as teenagers test their independence, they still need mum and dad.

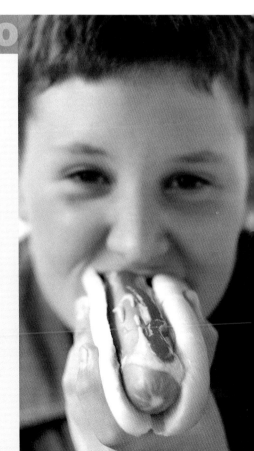

info

Teenagers at risk for Type 2 diabetes

A person with diabetes has elevated blood glucose levels as a result of a problem with insulin, a hormone produced in the pancreas. Insulin helps glucose (a simple sugar that comes from the food we eat) move out of the bloodstream and into the cells, which then use it as fuel. In Type 1 diabetes the body no longer makes insulin. (For more about Type 1 diabetes, see page 176.) In Type 2 diabetes, insulin is still produced, but is less effective in handling blood sugar. Being overweight often plays a role in the development of this condition, known as insulin resistance. Diabetes, insulin resistance, and being overweight all increase the risk for a teenager of developing heart disease, stroke, and kidney problems later in life.

Overweight teenagers
Once considered an adult disease, Type 2 diabetes is now starting to be seen among children. Although the number of children in the UK with Type 2 diabetes is small at present, many experts agree that Britain will be facing an epidemic within a decade because of soaring rates of obesity among children and teenagers. (For more about Type 2 diabetes, see page 21.)

Screening for diabetes
As many as 80 percent of children who have Type 2 diabetes are severely overweight at the time of diagnosis, which often occurs around puberty. Overweight children should be screened for diabetes, especially if there is a family history of Type 2 diabetes, the child has high blood pressure (a risk factor for heart disease), or the child has a skin condition called acanthosis nigricans. This condition – dark, velvety skin in the folds and creases of the body – is often associated with insulin resistance. Screening is important because a child with Type 2 diabetes may not have any obvious symptoms.

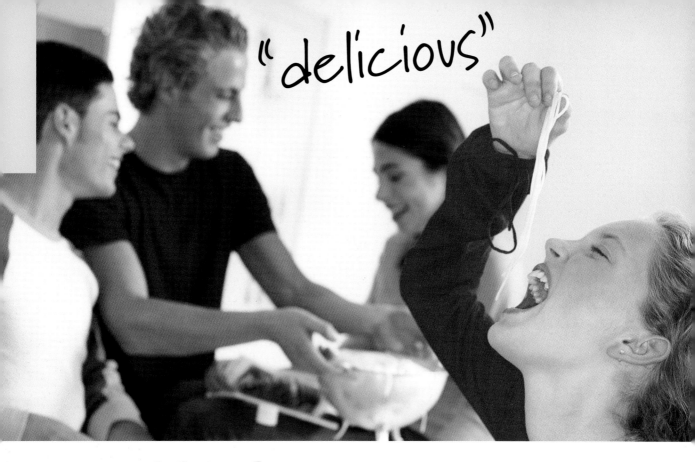

"delicious"

Nutrition for teenagers

Adolescence is a period of rapid growth that must be fuelled by additional calories. But not just any calories will do. Teenagers need foods that will build strong bones and healthy bodies for a lifetime.

The hard sell won't work

You know about good nutrition and what your child needs, but you can't force it on a teenager. However, while he or she may resist your efforts to promote healthy eating, remember that you're still in control of which foods you serve and make available at home.

Keep promoting good habits by eating well yourself and by serving family meals. Children who have regular meals with their family eat more healthily and even make more nutritious choices when they're away from home. Try to make arrangements so your teenager can be there at mealtimes. Providing structure like this can help your child stay grounded while so much else in his or her life is in flux.

Freedom of choice

While you're providing that overarching structure, it's also a time to be flexible and to give your teenager some freedom to make choices about food. Here are some good ways to involve your child:

- Your teenager's likes and dislikes may have changed over the years, so invite him or her to go shopping with you or make a list of foods for the dinner menu.
- Have your teenager help you prepare dinner once a week or take responsibility for certain tasks, such as making salad, on a regular basis. Your teenager will learn about making healthy food choices and, at the same time, he or she will acquire some basic cooking skills

Daily nutrition needs

On average, teenage girls need fewer calories than teenage boys. An active teenager (of either sex) will eat more, while a sedentary teenager will need less. As teenagers mature, their nutritional requirements become more similar to the recommended daily allowances for adults.

DIETARY COMPONENT	TEENAGE GIRLS	TEENAGE BOYS
Carbohydrates	246–280g	300–370g
Protein	41–45g	42–55g
Fat	61–70g	73–91g
Fibre	16–18g	16–18g
Total daily calories	1845–2110 calories	2200–2750 calories

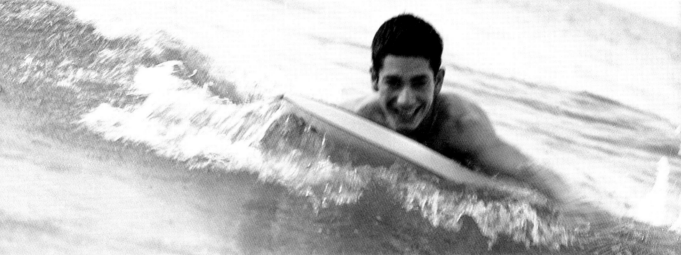

and gain an appreciation for what it takes to make a home-cooked meal. As a bonus, you'll get a little extra time together to catch up with each other.

- Occasionally, let your teenager take the lead by selecting the menu for a family dinner or even preparing the meal – with you as the assistant.
- Suggest that your teenager invites a few friends round to enjoy a special meal together. They can plan the menu and prepare it themselves. How about a pasta party? Here's a menu that's easy and fun: fresh tomato sauce with basil (see recipe on page 198) spooned over farfalle pasta (or any other pasta shapes), green salad, garlic bread, and Italian gelato or sorbet with berries.

Why teenagers need breakfast

While teenagers are in charge of choosing what to eat, they still should eat three meals a day. Yet many teenagers don't do this and may start the day on an empty stomach. Without a good nutritious breakfast, teenagers:

- are less able to learn;
- actually eat more calories during the rest of the day;
- are twice as likely to have diets low in iron;
- may have a higher body mass index (BMI).

On the other hand, teenagers who eat breakfast regularly:

- tend to eat healthier overall;
- do better at school and are more attentive;
- are more likely to participate in physical activities.

Ideally, your child would have time in the morning to sit down for a complete breakfast before dashing off to school. But many teenagers leave for school, or start school very early. So when there's no time for breakfast, do the next best thing by offering a variety of ready-to-eat breakfast foods.

Cereal is a quick meal and can even be eaten dry. Buy single-serving cereal boxes or make your own single servings, using polythene bags or containers. Choose lower-sugar, higher-fibre cereals or hot cereals that aren't loaded with sugar. Try pre-packing your own mix of nuts, seeds, and dried fruits that your teenager can grab on the go. Fresh fruit and yogurt are also good choices. Any breakfast is better than no breakfast, but to limit fat and sugar don't let your child get into the toaster tarts or Danish pastries habit. (See below for more fast breakfasts.)

The vending machine problem

If kids eat a healthy, sustaining breakfast, they are less likely to resort to eating at a chip shop or from a school tuck shop or vending machine – at least in the morning hours. High-fat and high-sugar snacks and drinks are available at or near schools all over the country. They appeal to teenagers for obvious reasons: they're convenient and inexpensive, and

they're tasty. But these kinds of foods don't provide much in the way of nutrition and they can be damaging to teeth. Many secondary schools in the UK have vending machines and the most commonly available products in them are higher-fat salty snacks, sweets, higher-fat pastries, and sugary fizzy drinks. Few of these machines offer semi-skimmed or skimmed milk, low-fat yogurt, fruit and vegetables, fruit juice, or bottled water.

Schools allow vending machines because it brings in much-needed revenue for them. Some schools also set up promotions with companies to encourage kids to buy more sweets or crisps in return for new sports equipment or books. Nutritionists and dietitians have been increasingly critical of these arrangements and the overabundance of unhealthy foods available in schools. While some changes are underway, it's likely your child still has easy access to these low-nutrient foods.

The solution is not an easy one because you can't follow your teenager around and supervise what he or she eats. But just as you've been doing all along, you can be sure that your child gets healthy, satisfying food at home. You can also encourage your children to pack their own snacks to get them through the busy school day.

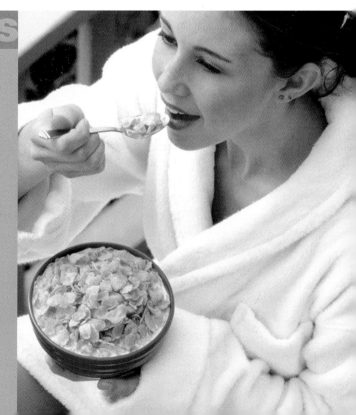

tips

Quick breakfast ideas

If your teenager doesn't care for typical breakfast fare, be creative by offering a favourite sandwich, a fresh fruit smoothie (see page 201 for some delicious smoothie recipes), or even leftovers. Here are some quick breakfast fixes to tempt your teenager.

- **Berry and cream cheese toastie** Layer cream cheese and sliced strawberries or other fresh fruit on wholemeal toast or a bagel.
- **Fruit and nut porridge** Add dried fruit or nuts to instant porridge.
- **Banana roll** Spread peanut butter in a whole-grain roll, pop in a banana, and sprinkle with raisins.
- **Breakfast wrap** Sprinkle grated Cheddar cheese over a corn tortilla, fold in half, and microwave for about 20 seconds; serve topped with a spoonful of tomato salsa.
- **Crumpet sandwich** Spread peanut butter on a toasted crumpet and drizzle with honey.
- **Fruity cottage cheese** Mix low-sugar fruit purée or compote with cottage cheese.

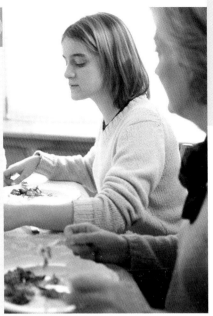

info

Why teenagers should eat family meals

What counts as a family meal? It's any time you and your family eat together – whether it's take-away food or a home-cooked Sunday lunch. Family meals are a comforting ritual for both parents and children. Teenagers know they will be fed and that their parents will be on hand. Parents enjoy seeing their children on this predictable schedule, which gives everyone a chance to catch up.

Teenagers who take part in regular family meals are:

- more likely to eat fruits, vegetables, and whole grains;
- less likely to snack on unhealthy foods;

- less likely to smoke, drink alcohol, or use cannabis or other drugs.

Strive for nutritious food and a time when everyone can be there. This may mean eating dinner a little later if your teenager is at an after-school activity.

Some teenagers may turn up their noses at the idea of a family meal, which isn't surprising considering that they're trying to establish independence at this age. It may be a challenge to get your teenager interested – or home in time. Try letting him or her invite a friend to dinner or prepare your child's favourite dishes. Above all, keep mealtimes calm and congenial – no lectures or arguing.

Temptations other than food

When parents teach children to eat healthily, the hope is that they will pick up the broader message – that their bodies need good care. This is important because adolescence is a time when it's common for kids to try smoking, drinking, and other risky behaviours. Some parents will just throw up their hands, believing there's nothing they can do about it. But this simply isn't true. With smoking and other dangerous habits, it's best to educate your child early on so the risks are clearly understood.

No smoking or drinking

Your teenager probably already knows that smoking can lead to serious illnesses like lung cancer and heart disease. Your teenager also probably knows that alcoholics often end up getting sick because of their heavy use of alcohol over the years. The trouble is that these health risks seem far off and not all that threatening to adolescents, many of whom feel invincible. You may remember this feeling.

Going on about long-term effects may be less successful than highlighting immediate effects. For drinking, there's the risk of being arrested for drunken behaviour or driving while under the influence of alcohol. A teenager who smokes may have difficulty recovering from colds or other respiratory infections, decreased cardiovascular fitness for sport, and – perhaps worst of all – bad breath.

Be proactive by teaching your teenager that part of a healthy lifestyle means avoiding cigarettes and alcohol. Share facts about substance use, but don't overdo the scare tactics. Most important of all, encourage open communication. Your teenager may not feel comfortable talking to you about everything, but if you are loving and welcoming you may be surprised how much your teenager may share.

Q: **My daughter and her friends say they smoke to stay thin. How can I get her to stop?**

A: Your best approach is to get your daughter to understand that using cigarettes as a method of weight control now could be the start of a lifelong addiction. Encourage her to stop as soon as possible. If she does need to watch her weight, help her do it through healthier means such as eating well and regular exercise. The best way to stop smoking is to gradually cut down the number of daily cigarettes. This might be easier if she has a partner. Maybe your daughter can encourage her friends to join her and they can kick the habit together. And if by chance you are a smoker, it's very important that you set a good example and stop smoking at the same time.

Helping 13- to 15-year-olds eat well

The early teenage years may be hungry ones for your child, especially during the periods of fast growth associated with puberty. To build strong and healthy bodies, growing teenagers need nutritious food, especially food that is rich in calcium and iron.

The effects of puberty

Before puberty, girls and boys have similar nutritional needs, but adolescence changes that for several reasons. The average girl hits her peak growth spurt at about 12, while the average boy doesn't reach that point until about 14.

Most girls in their early teens have had their first menstrual period, after which growth slows over the next year or two as they approach adult height. As girls are slowing down, the average boy is revving up. During puberty boys will need more calories than girls as they grow taller and more muscular, thanks to male hormones. Because each child will start puberty at a different time, calorie requirements will vary widely among boys and girls of the same age. As teenagers get older their nutritional needs start to resemble those of adults.

Differences for boys and girls

Just as daily calorie requirements differ for boys and girls during these years, so does the need for certain nutrients. Both boys and girls need iron, but menstruating girls – especially those who are very active – will need more, to prevent iron deficiency and anaemia. Boys and girls need calcium, but it is especially important for girls because they have a higher risk of developing osteoporosis later in life.

One-day menu planner **for 13- to 15-year-olds**

DAILY CALORIES
This plan will provide about 2100 calories.

Dairy products perform double duty in this menu. Milk, cheese, and yogurt are good sources of protein, with the added benefit of providing calcium. One thing dairy foods do not provide is iron, so look for alternative sources of iron, including iron-fortified cereals, pulses, and nuts.

breakfast
- 150ml (5floz) fruit juice
- 6 tbsp fortified cereal
- 200ml (7floz) semi-skimmed milk
- 1 slice of wholemeal toast with jam

FOOD GROUP	SERVINGS
carbs	3
dairy	1
protein	0
fruits	1
vegetables	0

lunch
- salad of 50–75g (2–3oz) tuna, 150g (5oz) pasta shapes, and 3 tbsp sweetcorn
- 150g (5oz) low-fat yogurt
- 150ml (5floz) fruit juice
- low-fat cereal bar

FOOD GROUP	SERVINGS
carbs	3
dairy	1
protein	1
fruits	0
vegetables	1

snack
- 250ml (9floz) milkshake
- 1 apple or other favourite fruit

FOOD GROUP	SERVINGS
carbs	0
dairy	1
protein	0
fruits	1
vegetables	0

dinner
- 150g (5oz) stir-fried vegetables with 50–75g (2–3oz) beef
- 4 heaped tbsp cooked brown rice or noodles
- 1 banana with custard

FOOD GROUP	SERVINGS
carbs	2
dairy	0
protein	1
fruits	1
vegetables	2

snack
- 1 slice of toasted wholemeal bread with cheese spread

FOOD GROUP	SERVINGS
carbs	1
dairy	1
protein	0
fruits	0
vegetables	0

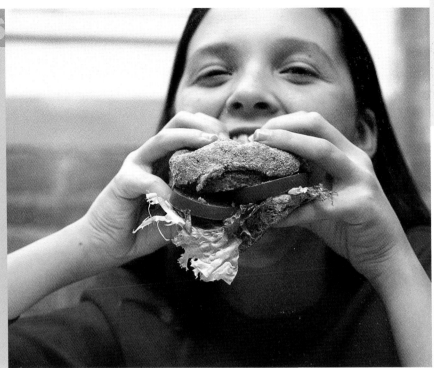

tips

Boosting iron intake

Here's how to ensure your teenager is getting enough iron.

- Use foods high in iron (meat, poultry, fish, fortified cereals, beans, tofu) in family meals, and be sure you have iron-rich or iron-fortified foods for snacking.
- To improve the body's absorption of iron, serve iron-rich foods alongside foods containing vitamin C, such as tomatoes, broccoli, oranges, and strawberries.
- Avoid serving coffee or tea at mealtime. Both contain tannins that reduce iron absorption. Milk can also interfere with iron absorption; if getting enough iron is a problem, avoid drinking milk when eating iron-rich foods.

Building healthy bones

During childhood and adolescence, the body uses calcium to build strong bones – a process that is all but complete by the end of the teenage years. Through the natural process of ageing, bones then become less dense. For some older adults bone loss is so great that bones weaken and break more easily, a condition known as osteoporosis.

When children get enough calcium and physical activity during the teenage years, they can start out their adult lives with the strongest bones possible. But a survey found that on average 24 percent of girls and 12 percent of boys aged 11–14, and 19 percent of girls and nine percent of boys aged 15–18, fail to get the recommended daily amount of calcium. Teenagers who smoke or who drink fizzy or caffeinated beverages or alcohol may get even less calcium because those substances interfere with the way the body absorbs and uses calcium.

Teenage girls may avoid dairy foods, a rich source of calcium, because they believe milk and cheese are fattening. But a 200ml (7floz) glass of skimmed milk contains only 66 calories and no fat, and it supplies 30 percent of the daily calcium requirement. In fact, people who eat diets rich in calcium weigh less and have less body fat: in one study,

teenage girls who had an extra 300mg of calcium each day (equivalent to 250ml/9floz skimmed milk) weighed up to 900g (2lb) less than girls who didn't get the extra calcium.

If, despite your best efforts, your teenage daughter adamantly refuses to eat dairy foods then she should eat calcium-fortified foods and may need a calcium supplement. You also might want to talk to your GP or a nutritionist. (For more information on calcium, see page 38. Find a list of calcium-rich alternatives to milk on page 132.)

Preventing iron deficiency

Both boys and girls need iron for a lot of body functions. When supplies of iron are low and iron stores are depleted, the body can't make enough of the red blood cells that transport oxygen to all the cells in the body. This is called iron-deficiency anaemia. Teenage girls need more dietary iron than boys because of blood lost during menstruation.

- Teenage boys should get at least 11.3mg of iron a day.
- Teenage girls need at least 14.8mg of iron a day.
- Athletes need more because iron is lost through sweat.

Iron deficiency can develop so gradually that you and your child may not notice the symptoms, the most common being fatigue and weakness.

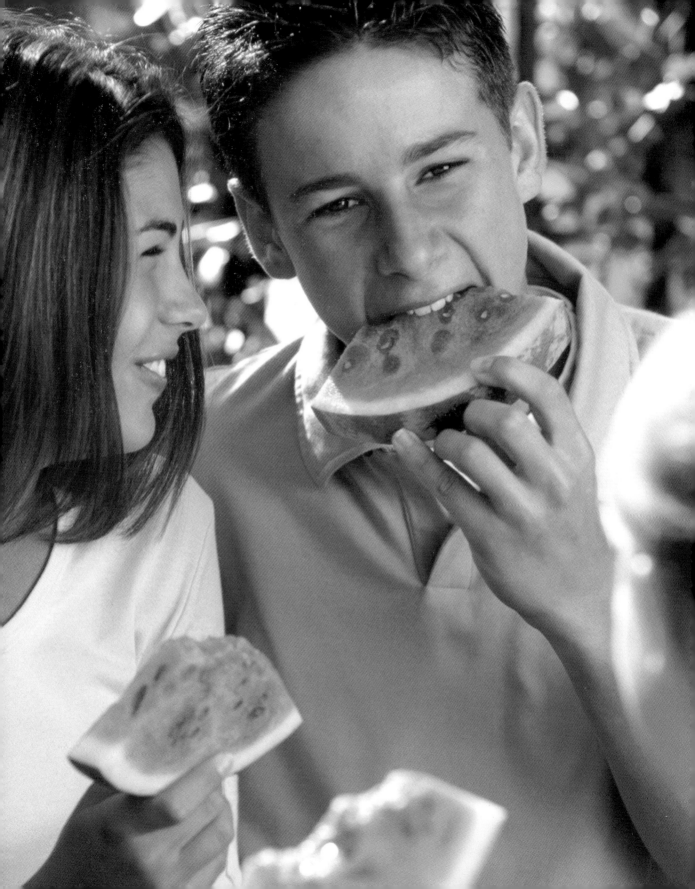

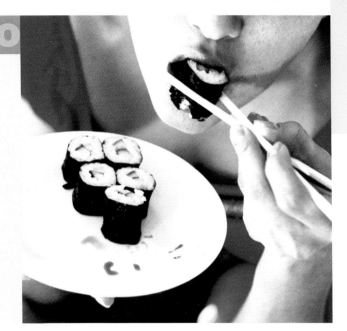

info

Different types of vegetarians

Many people who call themselves vegetarians are actually demi-vegetarians. They may have eliminated red meat, but still may eat poultry or fish. Even for those who have opted for a meat-free diet there are different vegetarian regimens:
- **Lacto-ovo-vegetarian:** eats dairy and egg products.
- **Lacto-vegetarian:** eats dairy products; no eggs.
- **Ovo-vegetarian:** eats eggs; no dairy products.
- **Vegan:** eats only food from plant sources; no eggs, dairy products, or honey.

Be wary if your teenager has self-imposed a very restrictive diet because being a vegetarian should not be used as an excuse to drastically reduce calories or cut out all fat. A teenager with an eating disorder may adopt a very restrictive diet and call it "vegetarianism" because that is considered socially acceptable and healthy. (For more information on eating disorders, see page 163.)

Going vegetarian

Teenagers often voice their independence through the foods they choose to eat. One strong statement is the decision to stop eating meat. This is common among teenagers, who may decide to embrace vegetarianism in support of animal rights, for health reasons, or because friends are doing it.

Avoiding meat may sound like a bad idea, but a well-planned vegetarian diet can be a very healthy way to eat, even for teenagers. Vegetarians often eat more of the foods that most teenagers don't get enough of – fruits and vegetables. A diet rich in fruits and vegetables will be high in fibre and low in fat, factors known to improve cardiovascular health by reducing blood cholesterol and maintaining a healthy weight. To support your child, the whole family might try to eat vegetarian at least one night a week.

Meeting nutrient requirements

The less restrictive the vegetarian diet, the easier it will be for your child to get enough protein and important nutrients. A vegetarian diet that includes dairy products and eggs (lacto-ovo) is the best choice for growing teenagers. A more

strict vegetarian diet may fail to meet a teenager's need for certain nutrients, such as iron, protein, zinc, calcium, and vitamins D and B_{12}. Calcium is a particular concern for any vegetarian who has eliminated dairy products. It's important for teenagers to understand which nutrients might be missing in their vegetarian diet so they can replace them. Failure to do so can lead to nutritional deficiencies.

Depending on the type of vegetarian diet chosen (see above) a teenager can miss out on important nutrients. Here are the ones they might be lacking and good food sources:
- protein: dairy products, eggs, tofu, pulses, nuts
- vitamin B_{12}: dairy products, eggs, and vitamin-fortified products, such as cereals, breads, soya and rice drinks
- vitamin D: dairy products, fortified breakfast cereals, margarines
- calcium: dairy products, dark green leafy vegetables, broccoli, chickpeas, calcium-fortified products including orange juice, soya and rice drinks, cereals
- iron*: pulses, whole grains, brown rice, leafy green vegetables, iron-fortified cereals and bread
- zinc: wheat germ, nuts, fortified cereal, pulses.

(*These foods contain iron, but are not as iron-rich as meat.)

The principles of planning a vegetarian diet are the same as planning any healthy diet: provide a variety of foods and include foods from all the food groups. A balanced diet will provide the right combinations to meet nutritional needs.

Variety and balance
Fresh fruit is an important part of a healthy diet, but restrictive diets that allow only raw foods or are limited to fruits or juices should be avoided.

Keeping 16- to 18-year-olds eating healthily

For most older teenagers dramatic growth has ended and they are settling into their new bodies. While taking on new responsibilities it's easy to overlook an important one: taking care of themselves with a healthy diet and lots of physical activity.

Guidelines for parents and kids

Older teenagers might now be driving cars and working part-time. They also may be learning to wash their clothes and manage money. Among all these new responsibilities is one that is very important but often forgotten: how to eat healthily – even when mum and dad aren't around. Many teenagers are fixing their own dinners, but are they preparing meals that meet their nutritional needs? This question takes on added importance if your older teenager is getting ready to leave the nest. Will the temptations of university life prove too strong to resist?

A varied and balanced diet

You know what your teenager needs, but how do you translate this information into guidelines your teenager can easily follow? He or she won't want to count percentages of this and grams of that. A simple approach is to share with your teenager the general principles of a balanced diet and the importance of eating a variety of foods.

The good news is that by late adolescence most kids are taking an interest in their own health. A parent can help by providing reliable sources of nutrition and health information, and encouraging a visit to the doctor to discuss any possible concerns. (See page 202 for a list of useful websites for nutrition and fitness information.)

Parental influence

Older teenagers need to understand nutrition and how to eat healthily because they spend more time away from home. With their own money and keys to the car, many teenagers have the funds and the freedom to eat as they choose. For some, this choice may be a huge fizzy drink and a bag of crisps for lunch. However, you still can have influence by following these guidelines:

- Make family meals a priority.
- Be a role model by eating well yourself.
- Keep the house stocked with healthy foods.
- Teach teenagers how to make healthy meals and snacks on their own.
- Be aware of your teenager's schedule.
- Without nagging, ask if they've eaten during the day and what they have had.

Beyond this it has to be left up to the teenager. Though it can be difficult for a parent to accept, it is now largely the teenager's responsibility to decide what and what not to eat. Hopefully the years of practising good habits have made an impact so your child will be ready when really put to the test: living away from home for the first time. (See opposite for tips on helping your child adjust to university life.)

What's in the fridge, mum?
Older teenagers often fix snacks and meals for themselves, so be sure there are always plenty of nutritious and tempting foods available.

One-day menu planner **for 16- to 18-year-olds**

DAILY CALORIES
This plan will provide about 2500 calories.

This menu is well suited for teenage boys, who generally need more calories than teenage girls. Cut down portion sizes or lighten up snacks for girls, to reduce calories, but try to keep the balance and the right number of servings of all the food groups. For very active teenagers, especially boys, add a morning snack and look for protein foods – which may better quell a voracious appetite – rather than piling on more pasta, potatoes, rice, and bread.

breakfast
- 150ml (5floz) fruit juice
- 2 scrambled eggs
- 2 slices of wholemeal toast
- 200ml (7floz) semi-skimmed milk

lunch
- chicken sandwich (2 slices of wholemeal bread, 75g/3oz chicken, 1 tsp mayonnaise)
- mixed salad
- 1 low-sugar low-fat cereal bar
- 150ml (5floz) fruit juice

snack
- 40g (1 1/2oz) cheese toasted on 1 slice of wholemeal bread
- 100g (3 1/2oz) grapes
- 200ml (7floz) semi-skimmed milk

dinner
- 225g (8oz) pasta with fresh tomato sauce (see recipe on page 198)
- 115g (4oz) chicken breast
- mixed salad with low-fat dressing
- piece of fruit or fruit salad

snack
- 3 tbsp cereal
- 200ml (7floz) semi-skimmed milk

FOOD GROUP	SERVINGS	FOOD GROUP	SERVINGS	FOOD GROUP	SERVINGS	FOOD GROUP	SERVINGS	FOOD GROUP	SERVINGS
carbs	2	carbs	3	carbs	1	carbs	3	carbs	1
dairy	1	dairy	0	dairy	2	dairy	0	dairy	1
protein	2	protein	1	protein	0	protein	2	protein	0
fruits	1	fruits	0	fruits	2	fruits	1	fruits	0
vegetables	0	vegetables	1	vegetables	0	vegetables	2	vegetables	0

Going to university

Even if your child was motivated to eat healthily and exercise when at home, university life can change all that. Unlimited cafeteria food, busy schedules, fast food convenience, and parties can add extra stones. The university years are prime time for older teenagers to gain weight and adopt unhealthy habits such as smoking.

Parents can't prevent teenagers from indulging in newfound freedoms, but they can offer some advice to their university-bound children. Explain that a lot of people gain weight when they go to university, but that it's possible to maintain healthy habits, even amid all of the temptations and pressures. Here are some tips you can give your teenager.

- Be smart about cafeteria eating by assessing all the options before choosing. Put together a balanced meal from the available choices.
- Be aware of portion sizes – it's easy to have seconds at a cafeteria.
- Don't study and eat at the same time.
- Keep a stock of healthy snacks, such as carrots, apples, microwave popcorn, and pretzels.
- Take advantage of campus exercise facilities – fitness equipment, swimming pools, and running tracks.
- Take the stairs, ride a bike, roller skate to class, walk or jog around campus – whatever way they choose, encourage them to be active while at university.

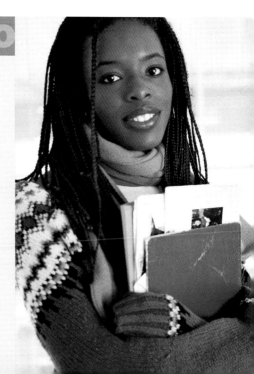

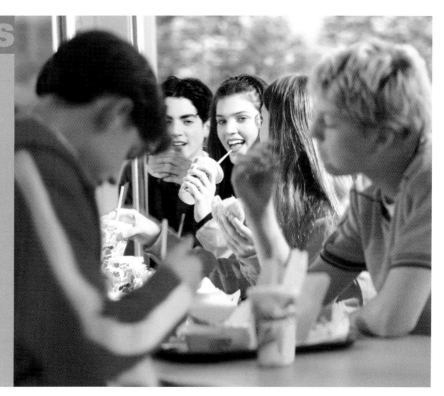

tips

Fast food orders

If your teenager is interested, offer these suggestions for eating lighter meals at fast food restaurants.

- Don't order "supersize" items.
- Order water, skimmed milk, or diet cola.
- Say no to mayonnaise and choose lower-fat condiments.
- Avoid extras such as bacon and more cheese.
- Check out the nutritional information for the items you're considering, so you can make an informed choice.
- Get a grilled chicken sandwich or a veggie burger instead of a burger or chicken nuggets.
- Try side dishes other than chips, such as a mixed salad, baked beans, corn on the cob, or some fruit.

Kids love fast food

Teenagers eat away from home much more than they did 30 years ago and fast food is often the choice. Fast food restaurants may be hard for your teenager to avoid because they often serve as hangouts. Some teenagers eat fast food because they're rushing between school and work, and have to grab something quick. Others may like it because it's tasty and cheap. But it's not low in calories or fat: a large burger meal with fries and a fizzy drink can contain more than half of the total daily recommended amount of fat and calories.

Teenagers who have fast food three or more times a week consume more calories and fat than peers who eat fast food less often. Eating fast food frequently also makes teenagers likely to drink less milk and eat fewer fruits, vegetables, and whole grains. Though you won't be able to ban fast food, you can try to help your teenager cut back.

Healthier alternatives

If you ask your teenager to eat less fast food, be sure to provide alternatives. If your child needs to eat on the run, suggest other restaurants that offer quick service and more nutritious food. Stopping at a sandwich shop or cafe for a turkey sandwich is usually a good alternative to a supersized cheeseburger. Even a slice of pizza and a salad beats the typical burger meal, especially if your child skips the fizzy drink or chooses water, semi-skimmed milk, or fruit juice instead. If a fast food restaurant is the only option, you can suggest ways to "lighten" their choices (see above). Another alternative is to pack a lunch or dinner for them to "take away". Keep healthy foods on hand at home, especially the ones your teenager likes, so he or she can put together a satisfying packed meal.

Your child may be less likely to go looking for fast food if family meals are part of the routine. Family meals tend to be more nutritious, but the positive effects of sitting down together for dinner go beyond healthy eating. (For more about family meals, see page 155.)

The teenage girl who diets

In a recent survey, six out of ten teenage girls said they would be happier if they lost weight. They thought thin girls were more popular and attractive to boys and had more girl and boy friends. Of those questioned, over two-thirds said they thought they needed to lose weight; however, only

19 percent were actually overweight. For a teenage girl who is overweight, taking action to slim can be a positive step. However, teenagers may try fad diets, fasting, and appetite suppressants, and may exercise excessively. These methods usually don't work over the long term and they can be harmful, especially to a growing teenager.

Girls who don't have weight problems may be dieting in pursuit of unrealistic weight goals. If your daughter is concerned about her weight, offer to set up an appointment with your GP. The doctor will check her height and weight and can calculate her BMI, to find out if there really is a problem. (For information about BMI, see page 18.) If your daughter is overweight, the doctor can suggest steps to take, which could include referral to a state-registered dietitian. If your daughter's weight is fine, the GP can reassure her that she doesn't need to diet to lose weight, and can reinforce the importance of healthy eating and regular exercise.

So many teenage girls choose to slim that it's worth opening a discussion about it with your daughter, even if you haven't noticed anything unusual. Talk about whether she has tried to lose weight and try to get a sense of how she feels about her body. What she says may surprise you. Even if your daughter is comfortable with her weight, you may hear about her friend who isn't.

Going to extremes

About five to ten percent of teenage girls exhibit some of the behaviours associated with anorexia nervosa (starving) or bulimia nervosa (binging and purging). A smaller percentage meet the stricter criteria for diagnosis of these eating disorders. Both disorders can be very harmful to a girl's health and can even be life-threatening.

A girl who has anorexia refuses to maintain an acceptable weight, has an intense fear of gaining weight or becoming fat, and has a distorted body image. She may refuse to eat with the family or join in other social activities. Bulimia is marked by recurrent episodes of binge eating followed by an attempt to make up for the overeating by purging, which may include vomiting and using laxatives.

Restricting calories during puberty can affect growth and delay the onset of menstruation. Significant weight loss after menstrual cycles have become established can result in irregular or absent periods. Get medical attention if you suspect your daughter may have symptoms of anorexia or bulimia (see below for a list of early signs). Treatment should involve a team of professionals to address the complex medical, nutritional, and psychological needs of a teenager with an eating disorder. Many teenagers with anorexia or bulimia may be dealing with depression or anxiety.

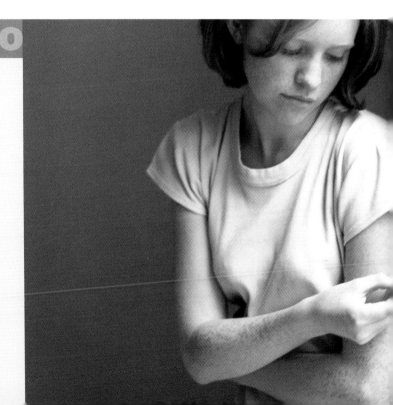

info

Signs of eating disorders

If your teenager has an eating disorder, the best approach is to get help early. With anorexia nervosa, watch for a teenager who:
- loses significant weight over a short period of time;
- seems to eat very little, cuts food into small pieces, or plays with food;
- wears loose-fitting clothes to hide weight loss;
- exercises compulsively;
- stops having menstrual periods.

Bulimia can be more difficult to spot, because the child will not lose a dramatic amount of weight. With this disorder, watch for a teenager who:
- shows a pattern of weight bouncing up and down (4.5kg/10lb up, 4.5kg/10lb down);
- spends a lot of time in the loo, especially after meals;
- eats a lot without gaining significant weight;
- exercises excessively to make up for overeating;
- has irregular or absent menstrual periods;
- has damaged tooth enamel from self-induced vomiting.

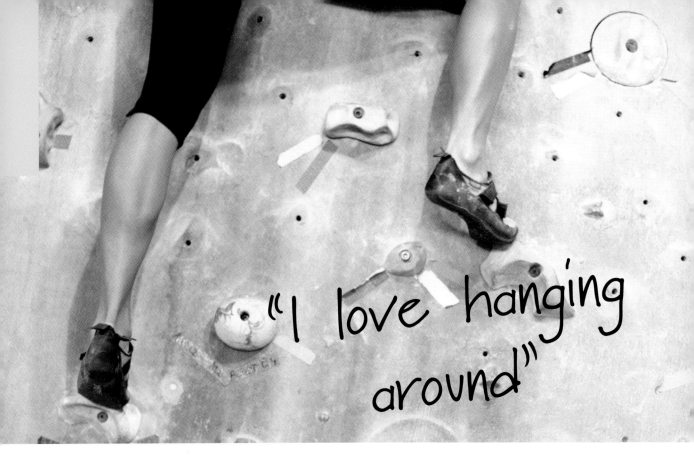

"I love hanging around"

Fitness for teenagers

It's a challenge to encourage physical activity in a technology-loving teenager, who has a mobile phone in one hand and a computer mouse in the other. But being active is important during these years.

Wired teenagers

Hey Prnts – RU sure ur tngr gts Enuf exercise? It's difficult to answer this when teenagers are spending so many hours a week online – many of them text-messaging friends in what looks like a foreign language. And while they are using the Internet, they are simultaneously eating, watching TV, and talking on the phone. If they get tired of that, they might take a break and play a computer game.

None of these pastimes requires much physical activity, yet teenagers need to move their bodies just as they did when they were younger. In addition to the health benefits of exercise, they need time to be "unwired" so they don't get in the inactive rut that many adults fall into. For younger children exercise often happens naturally, during break at school, by playing a team sport, or by cycling around the neighbourhood. But by adolescence, physical activity has to be planned and often must be sandwiched between various responsibilities and commitments.

How much exercise is enough?

The activity recommendations shift for teenagers, recognizing that they are moving towards adulthood and are no longer playing in the back garden. Teenagers should be encouraged to be active every day and to get at least three 20-minute sessions a week of more vigorous exercise. A teenager can meet this recommendation by running, swimming, playing football, or doing aerobics – or doing any other activity that gets the heart beating faster, quickens the breathing, and causes the body to sweat.

To be active every day, teenagers can do traditional exercises as well as everyday activities that get their bodies moving. During the week, a teenager might go swimming, take a long bike ride, and choose to walk to a friend's house instead of going by bus or car. Even activities that no one thinks of as exercise – such as taking the stairs, cutting the grass, or mopping the floor – can contribute to a more active lifestyle. In short, encourage your teenager to make a commitment to being active whenever possible.

Experts recommend that adults be physically active for at least 30 minutes a day, so teenagers can keep that in mind as a goal. But it's even better if they can exceed it. Talk about these targets and let your teenager decide how to achieve them. Keep your expectations reasonable, understanding that your child may have responsibilities such as studying that can't be eliminated from the schedule. But also encourage your child to take breaks during periods of inactivity – and to use free time in active ways.

Cool stuff to do

From the sedate to the wild, there's bound to be a sport or activity to suit every teenager's taste. Maybe your child doesn't like traditional sport – or is getting bored with the same old exercise programme. If so, try suggesting some of these alternatives to your teenager:

- paintball
- laser quest
- footbag
- frisbees
- dance (salsa, hip-hop, country, ballroom)
- water sports (swimming, diving, sailing, windsurfing, waterskiing, rowing, kayaking)
- fencing
- horseriding
- rock climbing (indoor and outdoor)
- snowboarding/skiing
- skateboarding
- skating
- outdoor sports (hiking, mountain biking)
- fitness classes (Pilates, kickboxing, yoga).

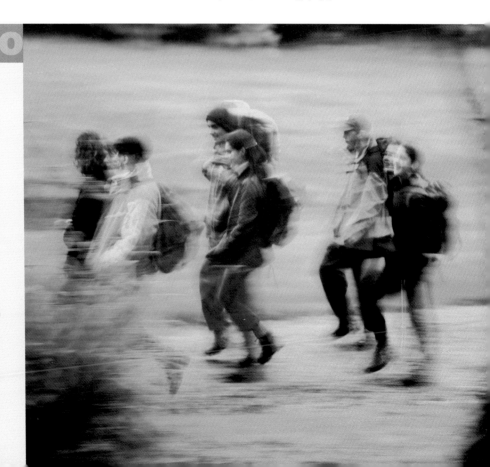

info

What is geocaching?

If your teenager is up for a high-tech treasure hunt, consider geocaching. This adventure sport, which is only a few years old, relies on global positioning system equipment to find "caches", which geocachers have placed in almost 200 countries. Getting to these caches can involve quite a hike, so you and your teenager will get a lot of exercise along the way. Adult supervision is recommended so teenagers don't get lost.

You never know what you'll find in a cache (CDs, a disposable camera, and small toys, for example), but they all include a log book so you can leave a record of your success. To practise proper cache etiquette, the finder may take something from the cache and should leave something for the next hunter. (For more information about how it's done, see page 202 for the website address.)

Motivating 13- to 15-year-olds to be active

By the time they reach secondary school, less than half of teenagers get regular and vigorous exercise. To encourage your teenager to be active, talk about the benefits of getting regular exercise and the best way to make it happen.

Getting teenagers off the sofa

What you say: "It's such a beautiful day, why don't you go get some exercise?" What your teenager thinks: "You're always telling me what to do." Whether your child complies with your suggestion or stays put on the sofa, this kind of approach will fall short because it doesn't acknowledge what a teenager wants: to be seen as an individual who can make independent choices.

One way to give your child some much-desired control is to let him or her decide how to be physically active. But before you ask your teenager for a list of exercise ideas, consider what will be practical, feasible, and affordable for your family. For example, if horseriding is out, let him or her know at the outset so you don't have an argument later. The possibilities for physical activity are vast enough that every child should be able to find something that sounds fun and interesting. (For a list of possible activities, see page 165.)

Don't be surprised if your child is most interested in the activities that friends are doing. Peer presure carries a lot of weight now, so seize the opportunity to hook a teenager on physical activity this way. Keep the group mentality in mind because it's likely to be an effective incentive. One good

Television hypnosis
Teenagers are spending more and more time in front of the "box" and computer. They often snack during these sedentary activities.

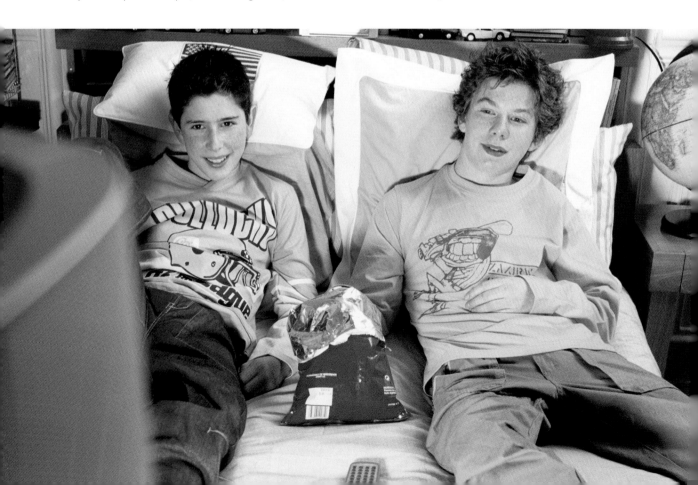

info

A sample fitness contract

Some teenagers may be receptive to this kind of agreement, where the expectations and responsibilities of both child and parent are clearly outlined.

Teenager portion

I agree to exercise three times a week for at least 30 minutes. I also agree to limit the amount of time I spend doing things that aren't active. They include:

- watching TV, a video, or DVD
- using the computer for fun
- playing video games

I will engage in these activities for a maximum of one hour on school days and a maximum of four hours at the weekend: no more than nine hours total per week. I can "bank" unused time for use later at a mutually agreeable time.

Signed,

_____
(Teenager)

Parent portion

In return, I will support my child's efforts to exercise three times a week. When needed, I will provide transportation to the swimming pool, park, or other recreational facility for my child and up to two friends. For agreed-upon activities, I'll provide the necessary equipment (clothes, shoes, protective gear). To manage TV time, I'll provide a TV schedule to help my child decide how to "spend" TV time. I'll also agree to pay for the rental of approved videos or DVDs.

Signed,

_____
(Mum or Dad)

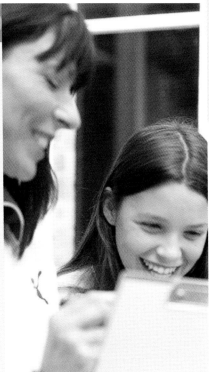

idea is to suggest that your teenager organize a group of friends to take a class or try a supervised adventurous activity, such as rock climbing, paintball, or laser tag.

Young teenagers love a chance to show their age and take on the responsibilities that go along with being older and wiser. Look for opportunities that will help boost your child's confidence and self-esteem. Consider letting your teenager work as a junior activities leader at a summer camp or assistant coach of a younger sibling's sports team. As a bonus, part-time jobs like these are active, which means that your child may get some exercise without even realizing it.

In addition to promoting regular exercise, parents need to limit the amount of time teenagers spend watching TV or playing video or computer games.

A parent-child fitness contract

If you and your teenager squabble about exercise, it can help to negotiate a contract. A contract sends two key messages: that you are serious about physical activity and that you see your child's input as critical. Be clear that the contract isn't intended as a punishment, but that it will allow both parties to clearly state their expectations and their responsibilities.

A contract should include the stated goal as well as the responsibilities of both the teenager and parent. Here's a step-by-step approach:

- Parent and child separately create a list of goals.
- Work together to negotiate mutually acceptable goals and expectations.
- Create a contract based on the agreed-upon goals. Try to be as specific as possible and take small steps towards progress. (See above for a sample contract.)
- Put the contract in a prominent spot, such as on the fridge door.

You also might want to include your own commitment to exercise as part of the contract – it will be far more effective as an incentive if you are setting an example. If you don't, your teenager will be more than happy to point out the contradictions in your behaviour.

As with any contract, the parent and teenager should be flexible and willing to renegotiate as circumstances change. Remember, the goal isn't the contract itself. It's the positive changes in your teenager's habits. At some point you might even agree that the contract is no longer needed because your child has adopted a healthier lifestyle.

Helping 16- to 18-year-olds keep fit

As teenagers get older their responsibilities increase and their free time decreases. And, like their parents, they may have little time to exercise. Parents have to take a back seat now and let their teenagers work at fitting activity into their schedules.

Busy lifestyles

Many teenagers are juggling part-time jobs, relationships, schoolwork, and many other activities. Meanwhile, they're thinking about the future and some may be filling out university applications. Their busy schedules rival those of their parents. The time crunch may lead

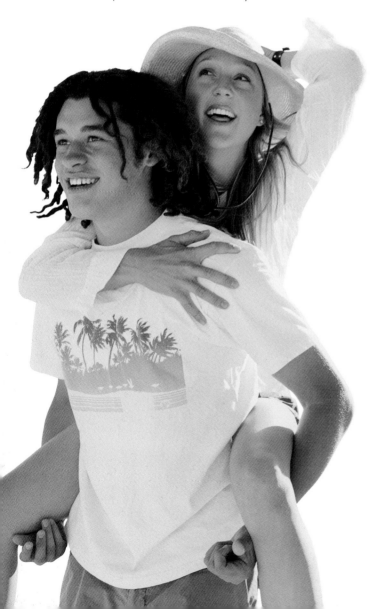

some teenagers to drop out of organized sport, if they haven't already. For sedentary teenagers the increasing responsibilities may become a reason not to be active.

If you have been preaching about the importance of fitness all along you may be pleased to discover your child seems to have got the message. In fact, older teenagers may be more receptive to what parents have to say about fitness and exercise – without any nagging some may even take the initiative to go for a run, have a swim, or join an exercise class. Though teenagers may not be swayed by warnings about their future cardiovascular health, they may be inspired by the immediate benefits of exercise such as increased energy, a feeling of well-being, reduced stress, and a firmer, fitter body.

As your teenager works to fit exercise into a busy schedule, you can still help in these ways:

- Continue to have an active lifestyle yourself.
- Plan active outings as a family.
- Fit exercise into your own schedule.
- Encourage your teenager to pursue lifetime sports, such as swimming, tennis, or cycling.
- As with younger kids, discourage watching TV or playing computer games.

A parent also can help by buying equipment or a gym membership, offering to be an exercise partner, or suggesting exercise videos or classes. Transportation can be an obstacle, so offer to drive your child or give permission for him or her to use the car.

A part-time job can also help a sedentary teenager be more active: many jobs involve physical work, and even those that don't will reduce the amount of time that is spent passively at home. Be aware though that a working teenager may turn to fast food when hunger strikes, so be sure to help them fit healthy meals into their schedule.

New partners
As they near adulthood, older teenagers still have an appetite for fun but also are taking on more responsibilities, including romantic relationships.

If your teenager has a job

Your child's job is your business, even though he or she is getting older. Help your child decide which jobs are worth applying for and in developing a list of questions to ask prospective employers. Consider the various reasons your child wants a job: money, work experience, or something to do. No matter what the motivation is, the job should not interfere with school. It's also important that teenagers have time to relax and meet basic needs like sleeping.

Once your teenager has got a job, monitor how it changes his or her eating habits. A teenager working long shifts might not get much of a chance to eat regular meals. The result is that the teenager might skip meals entirely or pig out after work, eating far more than he or she would normally have at mealtimes. At the other extreme, a teenager working in a restaurant may have access to free food, which can be a problem if weight is a concern.

Getting a part-time job
Working can be an enriching experience for teenagers as long as they still have enough time to study and to participate in school activities.

Q: **Should I limit the number of hours my 16-year-old son works?**

A: A teenager shouldn't have a job that interferes with schoolwork. It's also important for your child to have other interests and participate in sport or other physical activities. If your son's job is making this impossible, have him reduce the number of hours he works or suggest he stops working until summer.

If you and your son decide he can continue working during term time, here are guidelines to follow. They are intended for 15- to 16-year-olds who are still at school.

During the school year, a teenager should not:
- work before 7 am or after 7 pm;
- work more than two hours a day on a school day, eight hours on Saturdays;
- work more than 12 hours a week.

During school holidays, a teenager should not:
- work before 7 am or after 7 pm;
- work more than eight hours a day;
- work more than 35 hours a week.

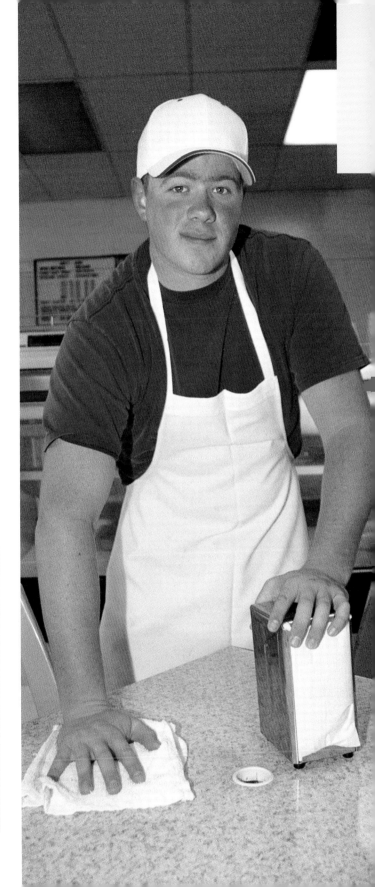

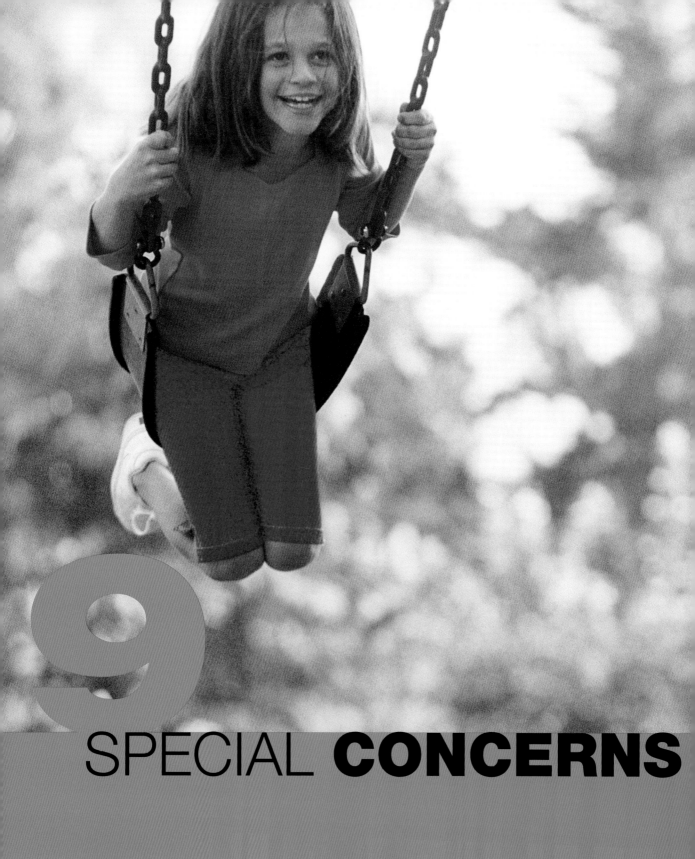

9 SPECIAL CONCERNS

Some children may face **nutritional and fitness challenges**. Whether they are gifted athletes or they face special **physical or medical needs**, parents have to look out for their **child's health** and well-being.

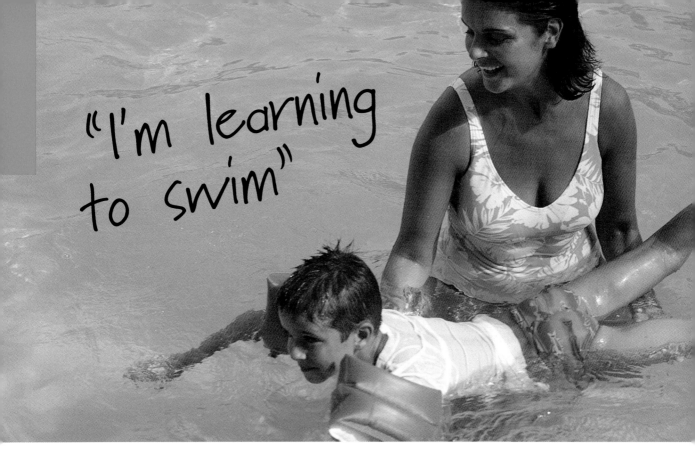

"I'm learning to swim"

Special challenges

Having a health condition can affect the way a child eats or gets physical activity. But parents can help their child be part of the action – from eating cake at a party to joining a sports team.

Before they play

If your child has a physical or health problem and wants to get active, the first step is to see your child's doctor, who will know your child's medical history. This should also be done before your child begins a new activity or sport. It's a good idea even if it's not required, because the doctor can identify any potential problems and also help to minimize the risk of injury.

Make sure children – especially older ones – know that the visit to the doctor is intended to help them participate safely, not exclude them. The vast majority of children, even those with existing medical conditions, will be approved for their sport or activity. For children with known health problems, the doctor may have to adjust medications or make suggestions about how to accommodate the child's participation in sport and other activities. (See opposite for information about some professionals who can be of help.)

The vital role of parents

Some medical problems, such as food allergies and the less serious food intolerances, affect a child's diet because the problem food must be avoided. Asthma, on the other hand, may affect the way a child gets exercise, with certain sports being better choices than others. And some conditions, such as diabetes, require special attention to both nutrition needs and physical activity.

Whatever the circumstances, all children benefit from eating well and being active, and parents play a key role in helping their child do both. It may mean choosing the right sport for a child who has attention problems or being sure a child who has diabetes gets a snack during the football match.

When a child feels different

A child with a medical problem may feel self-conscious and worry about not being like everyone else. Even if the only outward sign is that your child must visit the school nurse for medication, other kids will notice and wonder why. Reassure your child that everyone is different in some way. Here are some ways to help your child feel better about a condition that requires special attention.

- Educate your child. A child who's educated about a health condition is better equipped to handle situations that arise, including questions from peers about why he or she is taking medicine or eating a special diet. Role playing may help reinforce what your child has learned.
- Make a "crib sheet". Type up a list if your child finds it difficult to remember special instructions, such as foods to avoid or when to take medication. You may want to laminate the sheet so it won't be torn.

- Inform teachers. Your child's teacher can keep an eye on your child and watch for teasing or bullying from other pupils.
- Be supportive. Children with special needs will feel different, so it's important for parents to let them know they are loved for who they are.

It's important for all children to be active, so don't let your child's special needs be an excuse for being sedentary. Keep in mind that there are many ways to be active and you can tailor the type of activity to suit your child's interests and abilities. Young children benefit from adult-led activities, and with the help of your GP you can decide the best approach. Time for free play, where your child is left to his or her own devices, is a great way to let your child set the pace. Refer to the age-specific chapters for ideas, although do remember that appropriate activities may vary depending on your child's situation.

As children get older parents also might want to search out sports programmes and holiday camps designed just for their child. There are a great many organizations and professionals who can help you find the right programme to meet your child's individual needs. (See page 202 for useful names and addresses.)

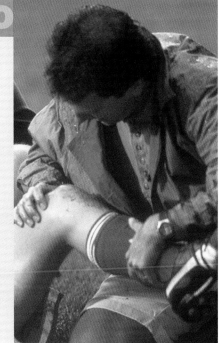

info

Professionals who can help

There is a variety of health professionals who can help you and your GP address the particular nutritional and physical needs of your child. They include:

State-registered dietitians: can offer reliable information on a healthy diet, menu plans, portion control, and special dietary considerations.

Occupational therapists: help improve skills needed to do everyday things, including learning and playing; can provide adaptive equipment so kids with special needs can be active.

Orthopaedic surgeons: treat sports injuries, especially serious ones that require surgery; also play an important role in the care of children who have physical disabilities.

Physiotherapists: help improve flexibility, joint mobility, and muscle strength; can work with children who are recovering from sports injuries or with children who have physical conditions that limit them.

Sports medicine doctors: specialize in the care of athletes during all phases of training and competition; in addition to treating injuries, can help athletes optimize performance.

Allergists/immunologists: test for and treat allergies, including food allergies and sensitivities.

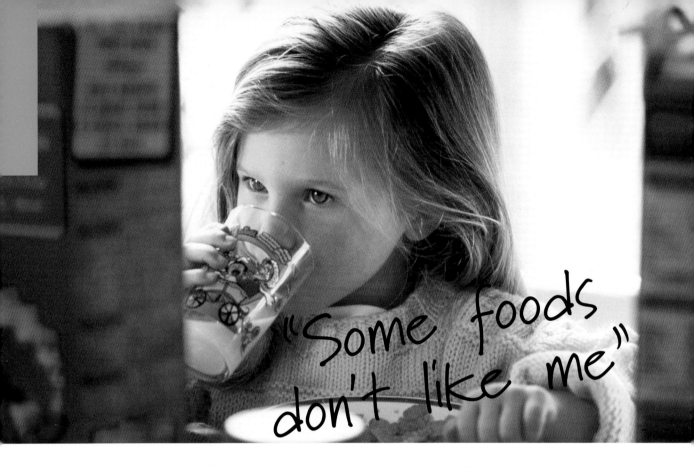

"Some foods don't like me"

The child with food allergies

Food allergies, and the less serious food sensitivities and intolerances, are increasingly common problems among children. But they rarely have an impact on a child's overall nutrition.

Allergic to food

When a child has a food allergy, the body treats a food as a foreign substance, triggering an allergic reaction that can affect the skin, respiratory system, cardiovascular system, and gastrointestinal tract. Symptoms range in severity from a mild case of hives to a life-threatening anaphylactic reaction (see opposite). Foods that most commonly cause allergies are:

- peanuts and other nuts
- seafood, especially shellfish
- milk, particularly cow's milk
- eggs
- soya
- gluten (eg wheat and oats).

The chances of having a food allergy are increased if a child is exposed to these allergenic foods too early in life or if a parent or sibling has a food allergy. (See page 79 for more about this.) In the UK, it is estimated that one to two percent of children suffer from food allergy. Peanut allergies have become a particular problem because peanuts are so commonly found in many commercially prepared foods.

With any food allergy, the best strategy is to avoid the problem food. Improved food labelling laws and the variety of alternatives on the market make it possible to do this, while still getting the nutrients required. For example, if your child has an allergy to cow's milk there are alternative sources of calcium, such as calcium-fortified orange juice.

Q: How can my child deal with food allergies or intolerances at school?

A: About 20 percent of children with food allergies or intolerances will have a reaction at school. Although most of these reactions are not serious – a rash, for example – some children will have difficulty breathing and, in some cases, the reactions may be life-threatening. As a matter of routine, all schools must have a clear procedure for calling an ambulance.

Talk with your child's doctor about developing an emergency treatment plan that can be shared with the school staff. Note, though, that while school staff have a professional duty to safeguard the health and safety of pupils, this does not mean they have a duty to administer medication. However, the staff may voluntarily undertake this responsibility and receive training that will enable them to do so.

Sensitivities or intolerances

Food sensitivities, which are also called food intolerances, can be confused with food allergies, but in general they are less serious and can be managed more easily. It doesn't mean your child is allergic to a particular food, but he or she can still experience uncomfortable symptoms. Lactose intolerance, for example, means that a person has trouble digesting lactose, a type of sugar found in dairy foods. The child with lactose intolerance may complain about wind, bloating, or diarrhoea after drinking milk or eating cheese.

What parents can do

If your child must avoid certain foods because of allergies or sensitivities, discuss your child's nutrition with your GP or a state-registered dietitian. If you are concerned that your child is missing out on important nutrients, ask about giving your child a vitamin or mineral supplement. When they are old enough, teach children with allergies or food sensitivities to make good decisions for themselves. For instance, your child shouldn't share or swap food with a friend. You also can teach your child to read food labels and ingredient lists, and ask questions about what's in a dish.

Talk with the doctor about what to do if your child has a serious allergic reaction. The doctor may recommend keeping adrenaline medication on hand and carrying an emergency injection kit. Your GP will help you learn when it's appropriate to give these medications, and at what age you can teach your child to take emergency measures for himself or herself. As an added precaution, make sure your child has a medic alert bracelet and wears it at all times.

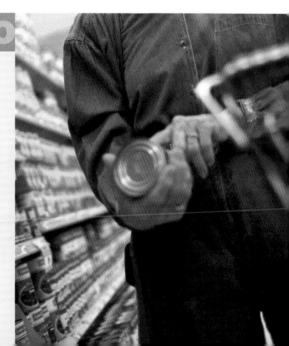

What is anaphylaxis?

A severe allergic reaction to a food or other allergens can result in anaphylaxis, or anaphylactic shock. This is a sudden, life-threatening reaction that can cause one or more of the following symptoms:

- tingling around the mouth
- tightness in the throat
- feeling of fear
- hives and flushing
- wheezing or other breathing difficulty
- nausea and vomiting
- low blood pressure and rapid heartbeat.

If the allergic reaction progresses, the child could lose consciousness. If you suspect that your child is suffering anaphylactic shock, summon an ambulance immediately.

When your child has a food allergy that can trigger anaphylaxis, prevention is the key. Be sure to read all food labels and teach your child to be vigilant about avoiding the problem food. You'll also want to be sure that family members, teachers, babysitters, childminders, and anyone else who cares for your child know about the food allergy and what to do if a reaction occurs.

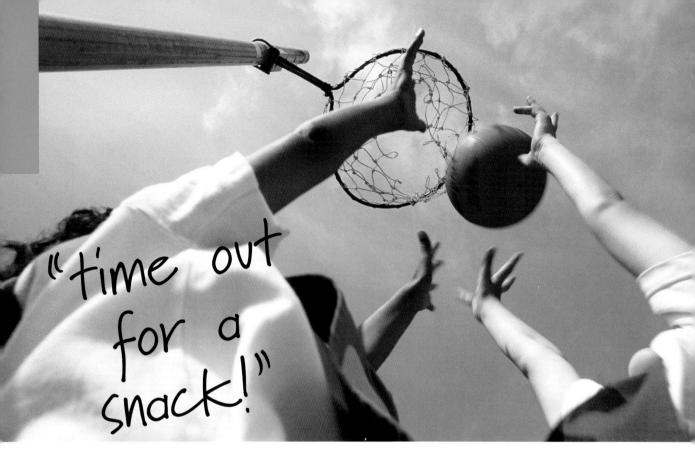

"time out for a snack!"

The child with diabetes

A person with Type 1 diabetes no longer produces insulin, which is needed to turn food into energy. There are special considerations for kids with Type 1 diabetes when it comes to eating and exercise.

Managing diabetes

Without the hormone insulin, the body can't use glucose from the bloodstream as it should. Glucose, a simple sugar that comes from the food we eat, is used to fuel our bodies. Fortunately, children with Type 1 diabetes can meet their insulin needs through injections with a needle and syringe or an injection pen. This insulin replacement can help keep a diabetic child's body functioning properly.

Children with diabetes need to be more aware of what they eat, how much they eat, and when they eat than other children. They also need to monitor their blood sugar levels regularly. A child with diabetes will work with a diabetes specialist to learn how to balance diet, exercise, and insulin

intake. There's no single management plan that is ideal for everyone. The plan needs to be personalized, based the individual needs of the child and of the child's family.

Nutrition needs

Just like all children, those with diabetes need a balanced diet that includes all the food groups (see page 40). However, special attention should be given to the amounts and types of carbohydrates in foods because carbohydrates are primarily responsible for the rise in blood sugar that occurs after eating. Control of blood sugar depends on the successful balancing of food (especially carbohydrate) intake with insulin dosage and physical activity. Children with diabetes and their parents may face a number of challenges in achieving this balance, particularly as the child gets older and spends more time away from home.

Parents should make sure that adults who will be supervising their child, including teachers, sports coaches, and other parents, understand the importance of following the child's meal and snack schedule. They also should know how to deal with hypoglycaemia (see below).

Many adults believe that sugary foods are completely forbidden for people with diabetes. In fact, most nutrition management plans for children with diabetes permit limited intake of these foods. Allowing a piece of cake or some ice cream at a birthday party can help prevent a child with diabetes from feeling deprived or different from peers, an important consideration in helping a child cope with the condition. Newer ways to give insulin, such as the injection pen, also give a child more confidence.

Exercise issues

While some precautions are necessary, children with Type 1 diabetes can exercise safely and should be encouraged to participate in physical activities appropriate for their age. In fact, maintaining physical fitness is a key factor in the management of diabetes. Regular exercise improves the body's response to insulin and can help a person have better control of the condition. Also, regular exercise helps all children maintain a healthy weight, which reduces the risk of heart disease in adulthood. This is especially important for children with diabetes since diabetes in itself is a risk factor for heart disease.

One aspect of your child's diabetes management plan should cover how to make adjustments for activity that help prevent hypoglycaemia. Talk to your child's diabetes specialist about adjusting insulin doses and adding extra carbohydrate snacks during times of increased activity. Good choices for snacks include fruit juice, low-fat and low-sugar cereal and muesli bars, and fruit.

Be sure you tell school staff – nurse, teachers, and sports coaches – about your child's condition and what should be done in case of emergency. Also, your child should wear a medic alert bracelet.

Type 2 diabetes

The management of Type 1 diabetes differs from Type 2 diabetes, where being overweight and sedentary often play a role. Previously called adult-onset diabetes, Type 2 is becoming increasingly common in children. (For more about Type 2 diabetes, see page 21.)

info

What is hypoglycaemia?

Low blood sugar, or hypoglycaemia, is more likely to occur when a person with diabetes misses a meal, eats less, or exercises more than usual. It can also occur when too high a dose of insulin is taken. Common symptoms are:
- hunger
- jitteriness and shaking
- weakness or drowsiness
- dizziness
- sweating
- headache
- glazed eyes.

If hypoglycaemia is not treated, the person could become confused or even lose consciousness.

The treatment for hypoglycaemia is to raise blood sugar levels quickly by giving carbohydrate-rich foods and other sources of sugar, such as a sugary drink, fresh fruit juice, honey or jam, or a mini chocolate bar. It's important not to send a child who is hypo unaccompanied to get sugary food; always make sure the child is with someone.

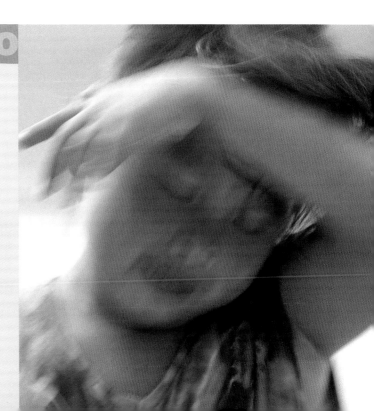

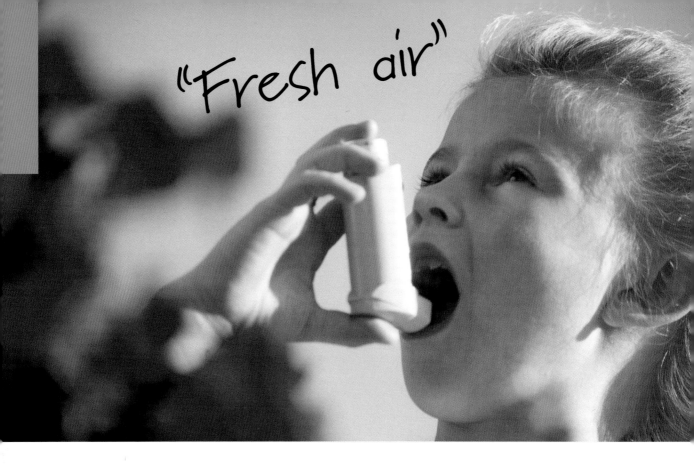

"Fresh air"

Helping all children be active

There are numerous conditions that can affect a child's ability to exercise and play sport. Two of the most common are asthma and Attention Deficit Hyperactivity Disorder (ADHD).

The child with asthma

When someone has asthma certain triggers, such as allergies or respiratory infections, cause airways in the lungs to narrow, making it more difficult to breathe. Symptoms are wheezing, coughing, chest tightness, and shortness of breath.

You might think that a child with a breathing problem shouldn't exercise, but for many children with asthma regular exercise is beneficial because it improves lung capacity and overall fitness. If children with asthma don't exercise, being out of shape can make them more prone to breathing problems. Inactivity also increases the risk that a child will be overweight, which can make asthma symptoms worse.

If your child has asthma you should first talk with your child's doctor about exercise so that all the proper precautions can be taken to make physical activity safe and enjoyable.

Getting medication right

As part of an asthma management plan, most kids use inhaled medicine to relieve symptoms during an asthma attack. Your child may be on other medications as well. In any case, before your child takes up a new sport or activity you'll want to talk with your GP about whether these medications or dosages need to be adjusted. Never adjust the medications yourself without consulting the doctor first.

You'll also want to inform sports coaches about your child's asthma, so they are aware and know what do to in the event of an attack. Your child also should know how to handle an attack. Tell the child to stop, rest, and use an inhaler if needed. See your GP if symptoms are severe, last longer than usual, or don't respond to the inhaled medicine.

While exercise generally benefits children with asthma, it can trigger asthma symptoms in some. This is more likely to occur in cold, dry air, so wearing a hat and scarf may help to reduce the chance of an attack. Using an inhaler before any physical activity may also help.

Appropriate sports

Many professional athletes have overcome asthma to excel in a variety of sports. For a few children, some sports may not be feasible so they should choose one that they can participate in despite their asthma. Sports that require sustained activity, such as distance running, basketball, and football, may be too much of a challenge for some children with asthma. Better alternatives include cricket, gymnastics, and short-distance track and field events, because they require shorter bursts of energy. For a child with asthma, swimming is often an excellent choice because the warm, moist air at indoor pools makes it easier to breathe.

The child with ADHD

Many children with Attention Deficit Hyperactivity Disorder (ADHD) are easily distracted and impulsive and have trouble interacting with their peers, so their parents may think they would not do well at sport. But under the right conditions, sports participation can help a child with ADHD gain more control over his or her body and improve social skills.

Children with ADHD may face obstacles in sports participation, similar to those they face in the classroom or at home. They may be careless and take unnecessary risks with themselves or their teammates, or they may be less attentive and be injured by a ball or other player. But finding the right sport – with the right amount of supervision – can boost self-esteem, help them make friends, and help them learn control as they channel energy in a positive direction.

Choosing the right activity
Individual sports, such as martial arts, dancing, tennis, and swimming, are a good choice for children with ADHD because they often get more attention from sports coaches and can improve body awareness.

What parents should do

Safety is a key concern for children with ADHD. They may need more supervision, especially when using sports equipment – from cricket bats to balance beams. You might feel a bit uncomfortable drawing attention to your child's ADHD, but it's a good idea to talk with coaches about your child's needs. With the right help your child can benefit from team sports and the camaraderie of being on the team.

You should attend practices and competitions. Work with your child on waiting his or her turn, following directions, and practising good sportsmanship. Just learning these basics is a significant achievement that will spill over into other areas, making the child feel more confident and liked by friends.

While not every child with ADHD needs medication, it can help some kids be more focused. If your child takes medicine, ask your GP if the dosage should be adjusted. A child who is less distracted can learn better, both in the classroom and on the playing field.

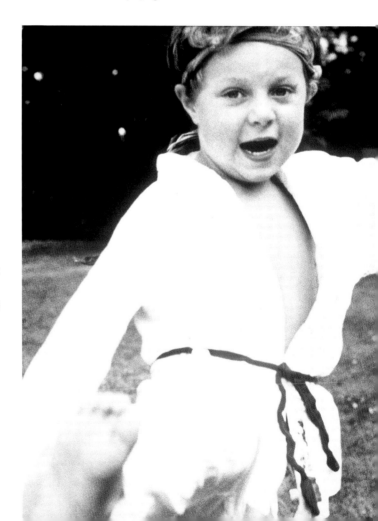

The child with special needs

Activity benefits children with disabilities. It improves their general health and they can gain flexibility, strength, and confidence, all of which can improve their present and future quality of life.

Overcoming barriers

Children with special needs can enjoy the power and the pleasure of physical activity. Just consider the wheelchair athlete who is adept enough to make a basket or the Special Olympian who runs across the finish line all smiles.

There are many physical, medical, and developmental problems that can create barriers to activity, but nearly all children can and should find ways of being active. Some disabilities that can affect a child's ability to exercise are: brain or spinal cord injuries; cerebral palsy and other birth defects; developmental disabilities; hearing and visual impairments; heart problems; decreased muscle tone); muscular dystrophy; and seizure disorders.

Exercise helps a child with muscular dystrophy maintain muscle strength for as long as possible. Staying active is also important for a child in a wheelchair, who may gain weight easily. Being overweight can compound the child's health problems and make day-to-day care more difficult. For a child with juvenile rheumatoid arthritis, physical activity has been found to decrease pain and improve mobility of joints. In addition to health benefits, children with special needs get an emotional boost as they feel a sense of accomplishment and – maybe for the first time – the thrill of victory.

Professional advice

Parents of children with health problems or disabilities may be reluctant to let their child play sport or exercise for fear that they will be injured or it will worsen their condition. But in most cases, doctors will permit a child with a health problem to participate in activities after having an evaluation, getting appropriate treatment, and taking safety precautions. Even then, though a child may be cleared for physical activity, some sports may be off limits. For instance, a child with an uncontrolled seizure disorder must avoid sports such as swimming or those where having a seizure would put the child – or someone else – at risk of injury.

"My pony doesn't know I can't walk"

Q: My child is disabled. Is a holiday camp a good idea?

A: A stay in an activity centre, specially designed to make outdoor leisure and recreation accessible, can be rewarding for a child with special needs. It's an opportunity to be with children who face the same challenges, and the child will get to enjoy being outside, participating in group activities, and having a chance to be more independent. A holiday camp also encourages physical activity, which may increase the child's confidence and desire to be active when he or she returns home.

To find a good holiday camp, get opinions from doctors and others who know your child, as well as parents of other children with disabilities. Charities and support groups are also great resources. Ask about care staff and special aids and equipment, to be sure the camp is able to deal with your child's special needs. Also make sure the camp is accredited by a reputable organization, which provides some assurance that the camp adheres to standards for safety, staff training, first aid, health care, and transportation. (See page 202 for more information.)

Many children and their families work with occupational and physiotherapists to improve flexibility, strength, and mobility. Therapists also can help parents select appropriate activities and make modifications, such as getting an adapted tricycle with a hand crank and foot straps.

In general, children with disabilities are encouraged to be physically active. Of course before exercising or trying a sport, you'll want to be sure that your child can safely participate in the activity. Talk with your child's medical and therapy team so they can recommend appropriate activities, as well as ways to accommodate participation and the precautions you need to take.

Special sports programmes

Children with special needs have more opportunities than ever to be active and involved. Most sports – even rock climbing and scuba diving – have been adapted to accommodate people with disabilities. For example, specially designed saddles allow children to participate in horseriding, which can improve balance and coordination. Goalball, introduced in the 1976 Paralympics, is specifically designed for people who have vision problems. The Special Olympics serves children and adults with learning disabilities, with free year-round training programmes. (See page 202 for some useful addresses and websites.)

tips

How parents can make the difference

Try these ways to encourage your child with special needs to be physically active:
- Teach your child to try for his or her personal best – not someone else's.
- Help your child make contact with other children with disabilities or chronic conditions through support groups or special holiday camps.
- Focus on fun, and send the message that just being active is the goal.
- Provide adapted sports equipment, such as a sports wheelchair, so your child will enjoy exercise and keep on doing it.

Praise children for their effort and commitment to a sport or activity and take notice of their achievements, even if they seem small. For example, if your child swims a lap just a bit faster or works extra hard in a therapy session, let him or her know that you're proud of them. Give them the sense of accomplishment that comes from knowing they did their best.

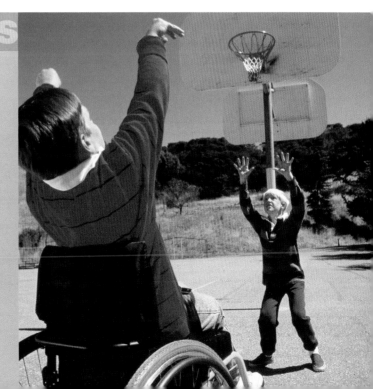

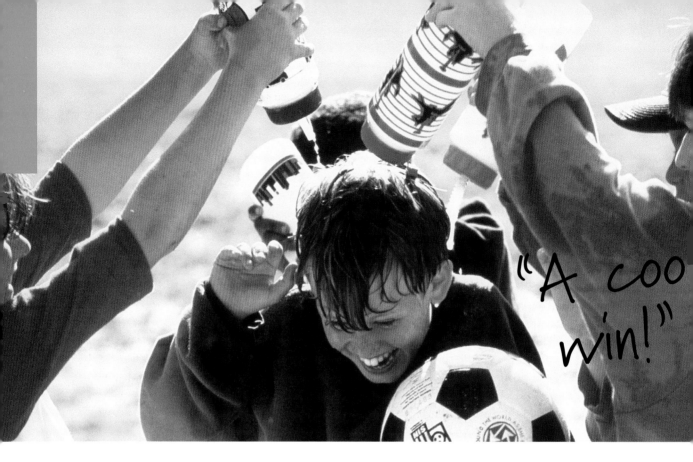

"A cool win!"

The child athlete

Very active children who excel at sports may seem little cause for concern. But they need special attention too, because of all that exercise they're getting during training and competition.

An athlete's special needs

Children and teenagers who are training for sport need more fluids and calories. In addition they run the risk of getting hurt, so parents need to know how to guard against injuries. Child athletes also need the watchful eye of a parent who can spot when they're over-scheduled, overdoing it, or taking health risks to improve performance (see pages 184–185).

Replacing fluids

Child athletes need to replace fluids before, during, and after sports participation. They are at increased risk of dehydration and may not drink enough to make up for what is lost during activity. Even mild dehydration can hurt performance, endurance, and concentration. And more severe dehydration could lead to heat-related illnesses, including heat stroke, which needs immediate medical attention. (See page 67 for a list of signs of heat-related illness.)

Fluid requirements depend on age, size, activity level, and climate. To be sure your child is getting enough:

● have him or her drink some water prior to match or practice time and every 15–20 minutes during activity;
● be sure the coach allows water breaks and that drinks are available during the practice or match;
● provide water bottles or sports bottles. If your child likes water ice cold, fill a plastic bottle and freeze it overnight. By the afternoon, it will be thawed but still cold.

Although water is the best choice for keeping your child athlete hydrated, drinks with flavour may be more appealing. Avoid beverages that contain caffeine, such as cola, and instead try a mixture of water and pure fruit juice or a sports drink. Both of these can be helpful during prolonged activity when children need to replenish their energy supplies and electrolytes from salt losses through sweating as well as fluid. Remember, though, that sports drinks contain sugar (and thus extra calories) so you may want to limit their consumption, particularly for a child who is overweight.

Food as fuel

The calorie requirements of very active teenagers can be astounding. In general, male and female athletes who train for more than 12 hours per week may need as much as 3000–5000 calories a day. Of course needs will vary based on age, gender, size, and their stage of puberty.

It may be worthwhile to keep a closer eye on your child's nutrition when he or she is in training. One strategy is to keep a food diary to look at total calories as well as how they are distributed among protein, carbohydrates, and fat. The proportions for an athlete are about the same as for a non-athlete. Some athletes, especially older teenagers who are strength training, may need more protein; however, high-protein diets or protein supplements are not necessary and may cause serious problems such as kidney damage. Calcium and iron also are very important (see below).

For those who need it, state-registered dietitians who specialize in sports nutrition can help assess your child's diet. They can tell you if he or she is getting enough nutrients and also how to make adjustments during off-season times if activity levels drop significantly then.

Regular meals are important

Athletes may skip breakfast and other meals because they're too tired or busy. Monitor whether they're skipping meals and put your foot down about it. Insist that your child eat breakfast every day. Yogurt with cereal or a piece of toasted whole-grain bread with an egg are excellent choices for fuelling up before activity.

The timing of meals and snacks is important to optimize performance. If your child is going to eat a full meal, serve it one and a half to three hours before match or practice time. During the practice or match, a snack may be needed, especially during all-day competitions. Prepare easy-to-eat snacks that can be packed in a sports bag. Half a sandwich, some fresh or dried fruit, and nuts are all good choices.

After the match, let your child athlete replenish energy reserves with a balanced meal. Family dinners can go by the wayside when a child is busy with sports practices and matches. When the evening is free, seize the opportunity to get the family together round the dinner table. At other times, consider having your evening meals a little later to accommodate the athlete's schedule.

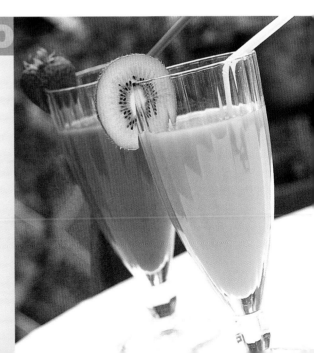

Calcium and iron requirements

Calcium builds strong bones, which are vitally important for athletes whose bodies endure increased stress and strain. Weakened bones are more likely to break.

Boys aged 11–18 need 1000mg of calcium a day and girls 800mg. To add calcium to your child's diet, serve calcium-rich foods such as milk and other dairy products, dark green vegetables, and calcium-fortified orange juice.

Iron-deficiency anaemia can hinder athletic performance and cause children to tire more easily.

One way child athletes lose iron is through sweating, so they need more to ensure peak performance and stamina. In addition, female athletes are at increased risk of iron deficiency due to the blood lost through menstruation.

Adolescent boys need at least 11.3mg of iron every day and adolescent girls at least 14.8mg. The best way to get enough iron is to eat iron-rich foods, such as meat, eggs, and dried fruit. Give your child an iron supplement only if the child's doctor recommends it.

Q: **How can I tell if my child is using steroids?**

A: These are some of the recognizable effects of steroid use/abuse:

- sudden increase in muscle size
- skin changes, including the appearance of stretch marks and worsening of acne
- excessive hair growth in females
- breast development in males
- male-pattern baldness (receding hairline at the sides of the forehead; loss of scalp hair at the crown, or top, of the head)
- violent behaviour and delusions

Preventing injuries

Many parents watching from the sidelines worry that their child athlete will be injured. Fortunately, there are some steps you can take to minimize the risk to your child. Choose a sports programme that takes injury prevention seriously. Coaches should be qualified first-aiders (ask to see their certificates) and there should be procedures in place for handling emergencies.

It's also important to educate your child about sports safety. Make sure your child:

- warms up appropriately;
- knows the rules of the game and is playing with teammates of a similar skill level;
- wears the right protective equipment for every practice and competitive event;
- plays on surfaces that are properly maintained and designed for the sport;
- participates in a variety of activities instead of focusing on one sport and performing the same repetitive motion over and over again.

Injuries do occur

Sometimes, despite taking precautions, a child is injured during practice or play. The three most common types of sports injuries in children are acute injuries, overuse injuries, and reinjuries.

- Acute injuries, such as bruises, sprains, and strains, occur suddenly. More severe acute injuries include broken bones, torn ligaments, and head injuries.
- Overuse injuries, which account for about half of sports injuries among secondary school athletes, occur when children perform repetitive actions that put too much stress on the musculoskeletal system. Such injuries are particularly problematic in childhood because they can

interfere with normal bone growth. Overuse injuries are most common in basketball, running, gymnastics, baseball, and swimming.

- Reinjuries are a risk when a child returns to a sport too soon. In addition the still-recovering athlete may be compensating for pain and weakness, which can result in additional injuries.

Recuperation time will vary depending on the injury, but never allow your child to "play through the pain". This may occur in professional sport, but it's not acceptable and often riskier for a child. Get medical attention for your child and follow the doctor's instructions about treatment as well as the advice about when it's safe for your child to resume participation in the sport.

Going to extremes

A child who is committed to a sport may start taking risks to improve his or her endurance and performance. Initially these behaviours may be mild enough to go unnoticed by coaches and parents. But they can lead children to take increasing risks to stay at the top of their chosen sport.

Losing weight

Wrestlers, gymnasts, skaters, and ballet dancers may feel pressure to weigh less. Some teenage wrestlers take extreme measures, such as fasting and trying to sweat off excess so they can make their weight class. Gymnasts, skaters, and dancers may be at risk of eating disorders because of the emphasis placed on thinness. For girls, this can lead to a condition known as the female athlete triad, a combination of three inter-related medical problems (see opposite).

If your child is involved in wrestling, gymnastics, skating, or ballet, be proactive by discussing weight issues with him or her. Watch for signs that your child is skipping meals, exercising excessively, or taking over-the-counter weight-loss products. Be sure your child knows that these practices are dangerous and that they may, in fact, worsen performance rather than improve it. (For more information about eating disorders, see page 163.)

Bulking up

Sports like rugby value strength, prompting some young players to turn to questionable supplements as well as illegally obtained steroids to bulk up for the rugby season. Many people mistakenly believe sports supplements are harmless because they're widely available and are often labeled as "natural".

Common sports supplements include:
- megavitamins
- herbs
- hormones such as androstenedione ("andro") and dehydroepiandrosterone (DHEA).

Despite the claims on their labels, these supplements are often ineffective and a waste of money.

It's easy to understand why young athletes are interested in sports supplements. Creatine, used by some well-known professional athletes, has been found to increase strength in some circumstances. But supplements should be considered unsafe for children because they're not regulated and have not been adequately tested, and often the effects of long-term use are unknown.

Steroids, on the other hand, are illegal without a prescription and are known to cause health problems. Steroid use in children may stunt growth, change behaviour, cause infertility, and damage internal organs including the liver and heart. Make sure your child understands the dangers of using steroids. Send a clear message that you disapprove and won't tolerate it. (See opposite for information about the signs of steroid use and abuse.)

Parental guidance

Everyone is looking for a magic pill, whether it's to lose weight or improve athletic performance. But such a miracle does not exist. Instead, parents need to teach their children that consistent training and healthy eating are the best and safest routes to excellence.

School and other children's sports teams ban steroids and performance-enhancing drugs, so using them could mean the end of your child's athletic endeavours. If you're concerned that your child may be using steroids, taking sports supplements, or trying dangerous weight-loss tactics, talk with the child's doctor.

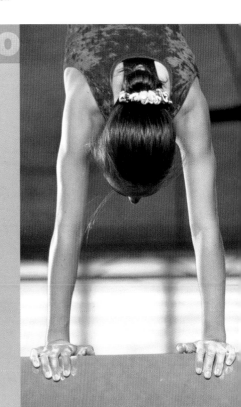

info

What is the female athlete triad?

A girl who feels pressure to stay small and slim for her chosen sport could be at risk for the female athlete triad, a combination of these medical problems:
- unhealthy eating pattern, ranging from dieting to a serious eating disorder
- cessation of menstruation
- weakened bones (osteoporosis)

Poor nutrition combined with excessive exercise causes hormonal changes that result in an interruption in regular menstrual cycles. The resulting low oestrogen levels can affect the girl's ability to absorb calcium, which is needed for strong bones. A lack of adequate amounts of calcium in the girl's diet compounds the problem.

Female athlete triad is common among gymnasts, skaters, distance runners, and ballet dancers, who may train and diet excessively to improve their performance.

Some young female athletes also may have a poor body image, which can be associated with a typical eating disorder. Because these problems occur while a girl is going through a key period for bone development, she may miss a critical opportunity to build strong bones. Even if the girl resumes her period and takes calcium supplements, her long-term bone health may be permanently affected.

Aside from missing menstrual periods, symptoms of the female athlete triad include fatigue, a decreased ability to concentrate, and an increased risk of bone fractures and muscle injuries. A girl who has the female athlete triad will need to cut back on her training and eat a healthier diet. To achieve this, she should work with her GP and a variety of specialists, including a nutritionist and a psychologist.

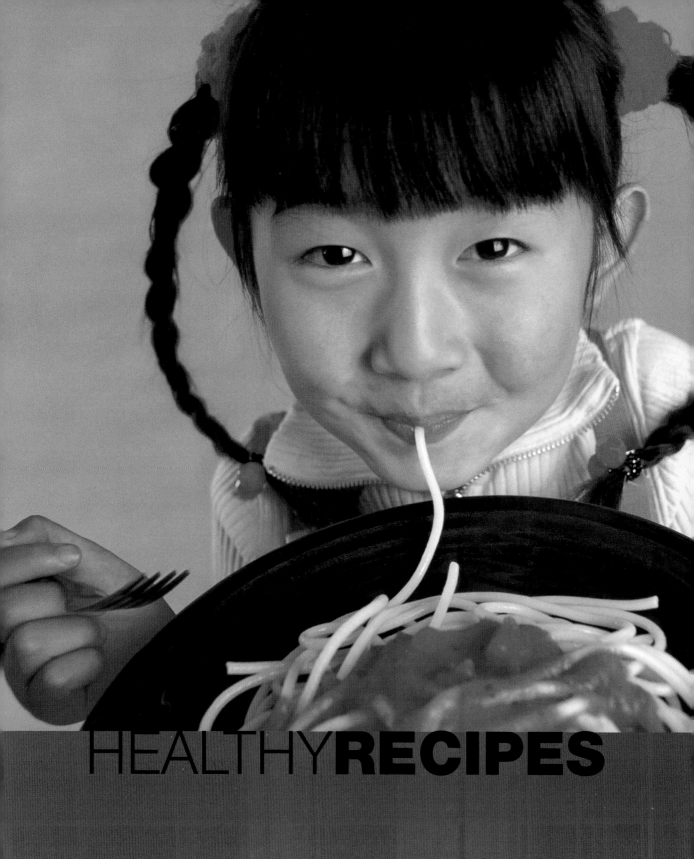

HEALTHY**RECIPES**

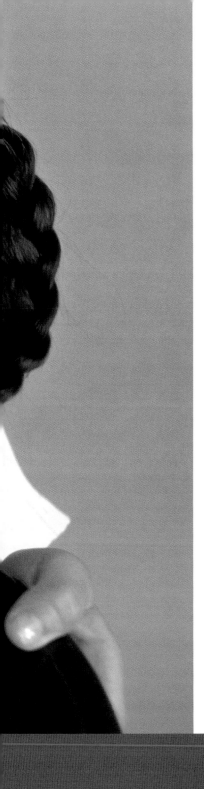

When your **meals and snacks** are home-made you **know what's in them**. Try these recipes if you'd like to bring **healthy, wholesome, and tasty** food to your family table.

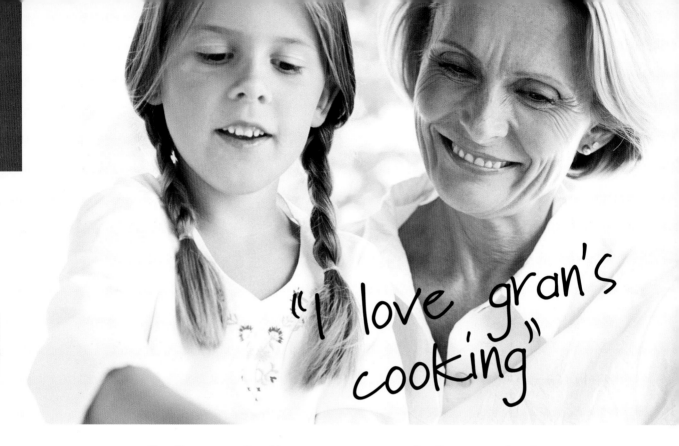

"I love gran's cooking"

Good food for good health

You don't need culinary training to cook nutritious meals for your family. Whether you're an experienced cook or a novice, you can improve the way your family eats. They'll benefit from your efforts.

Fitting in some cooking

Cooking does take time – time to plan meals, shop for the ingredients, prepare the food, and do the washing up. If you are in a pattern of eating out and heating up ready meals, it may require some juggling for you to fit home cooking into your schedule. But regular, nutritious meals for your family are certainly worth the effort – as the rates of overweight, heart disease, and diabetes climb, we're learning that a steady diet of lower-nutrient, higher-fat fast foods and take-aways may be contributing to this impending health crisis.

Feeding children is one of a parent's most important responsibilities. It is at once simple and complicated – as simple as making a cheese and pickle sandwich or as complicated as dealing with a child's weight problem.

The goals for all parents are to give their children nutritious foods and to foster healthy attitudes towards eating that will last a lifetime. Providing home-cooked family meals will go a long way to achieving these goals.

Plan meals in advance Having a weekly meal plan will save you from that awful feeling at the end of a long day, when everyone is hungry and you have no idea what to make for dinner. It may help to set aside time on the same day each week to draw up your menu plan. As you sketch it out, consider how you'll handle busy days when you and other members of the family have after-school or evening activities. Then make a shopping list and decide on the time when you'll go to the supermarket to stock up on the ingredients you'll need for the coming week.

Work ahead when you can If, for example, you know you want salad with tomorrow's dinner, wash the leaves tonight. Or buy pre-washed bags of salad. You also might marinate meats overnight, so they're already seasoned and ready for cooking. Saving that little bit of time can get dinner on the table with fewer last-minute hassles.

Make double batches for another day Soups and pasta sauces take considerable chopping and cooking, so why not make more than you need and freeze it? Then all you have to do later is thaw, heat, and eat. Or, if you prefer, wrap up the extra portion and keep it in the refrigerator, then eat the leftovers over the next few days.

The best choices

No matter how diligent you are, no family eats perfectly every day. Moderation is, of course, wise all the time, but one indulgent day or a holiday week will not blot out many more days' or weeks' worth of healthy eating. Good nutrition is an average and the aim is to improve how your family eats most of the time. Ask yourself these questions:

- What do you always have on hand for breakfast? For example, are the cereals loaded with additives and sugar or full of natural goodness?
- How do you cook foods? Do you often sauté or deep-fry or do you instead choose techniques that require little or no added fat? Do you boil vegetables in lots of water or steam them so they retain more of their nutrients?

- What kind of oil or fat do you use? Lean towards olive oil and other vegetable oils because fats such as butter, margarine, and lard contain greater amounts of less healthy saturated and trans fats.
- How much fat do you use? Regardless of the type, be sparing with fat when preparing foods at home. You often can reduce the amount of oil or fat in a recipe without affecting the taste, especially if you use flavourful oils. (See page 26 for more ideas about lightening up favourite dishes.) And if you use non-stick pans and cooking spray when frying or baking, you'll find that you need much less cooking oil or fat.

Recipe for togetherness

Not only can home cooking improve nutrition, it can strengthen family bonds and create a comforting tradition in your home life. Eating meals together provides a chance to talk and spend more time with each other. Preparing meals together adds another dimension. Children welcome the opportunity to get their hands dirty and play an important role in the creation of a dish the family will eat together. They may even want to taste whatever they helped make.

On the following pages, you'll find recipes for breakfast, lunch, dinner, and snacks. All are uncomplicated and call for easy-to-find ingredients. These recipes provide a variety of nutrients, but we have noted when the dish has a significant amount of particular vitamins or minerals.

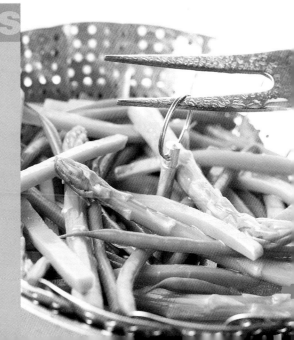

tips

Healthy cooking tips

- Leave skins on fruits and vegetables where appropriate, because much of their nutrient content is just under the skin and the skin offers valuable fibre.
- Prepare fruits and vegetables as close to eating or cooking as possible, to reduce vitamin loss. If not using immediately, cover and store in the refrigerator.
- When you cook vegetables in water some vitamins are released into the water; the longer you cook, the more nutrients are lost. So rather than boiling, poach

vegetables in the minimum of water or steam them for the shortest time possible.
- Poaching and steaming are great non-fat cooking methods for fish, as is cooking in the microwave.
- Little or no fat is needed when you stir-fry, cook on a ridged grill pan, grill, or roast meat and poultry. Roasting or grilling on a rack lets fat drip away.
- Most of the fat in poultry is in the skin, so to reduce fat intake don't eat the skin (you can take it off before or after cooking).

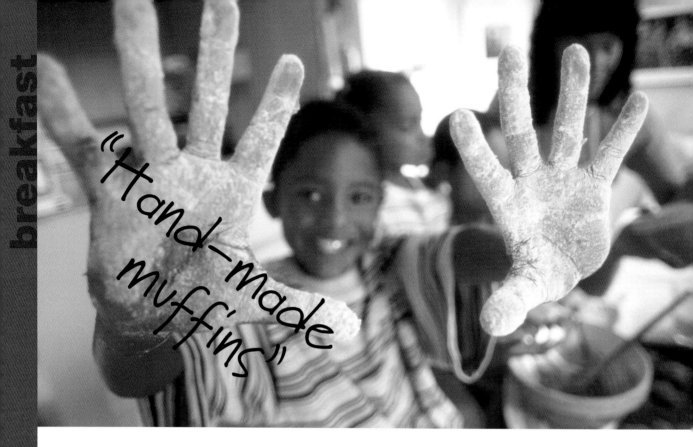

"Hand-made muffins"

Breakfasts to start the day

Hearty Swiss muesli

Makes 12 servings
(120ml/4floz each)

160g (5½oz) rolled oats

150g (5oz) raisins

480ml (16floz) semi-skimmed milk

240ml (8floz) low-fat plain yogurt

2 teaspoons honey

1 teaspoon pure vanilla extract
(optional)

340g (12oz) diced fresh fruit,
such as berries, apples, pears,
apricots, peaches, plums, melon

65g (2½oz) chopped walnuts,
flaked almonds, or chopped
pecans

● Combine the oats and raisins in a bowl. Add the milk and stir, then leave to soak for 30 to 40 minutes.

● Drain off excess milk, then add the yogurt, honey, and optional vanilla.

● Add the fruit and nuts, and mix together well.

● If not eating straight away, this cereal will keep in a covered container in the refrigerator for three to four days. You may prefer to add the fruit and nuts just before serving.

● This traditional Swiss recipe is a nice change from porridge or cold cereal. Feel free to adapt it to suit your child's taste by substituting different fresh fruits or omitting the nuts.

Nutritional analysis per serving	
calories	147
fat 1g (of which 0.5g is saturated)	
protein	5g
carbohydrates	25g
fibre	2g
minerals	iron, potassium, zinc
vitamins	A, folate

Food groups: carbs, dairy, fruits

Gingerbread muffins with fresh pears

Makes 12 muffins

2 eggs

120ml (4floz) buttermilk or soured cream

120ml (4floz) molasses or dark treacle

115g (4oz) unsalted butter, melted and cooled

115g (4oz) soft dark brown sugar

1 tablespoon grated or finely chopped fresh root ginger

200g (7oz) plain flour

1 teaspoon bicarbonate of soda

½ teaspoon ground cloves

¼ teaspoon grated nutmeg

¼ teaspoon salt

60g (2¼oz) crystallized ginger, chopped into small bits

Fresh pears, to serve

● Preheat the oven to 180°C (350°F, gas mark 4). Lightly grease a 12-cup muffin tray or use paper liners in the muffin cups.

● Beat the eggs in a mixing bowl. Stir in the buttermilk or soured cream, molasses, butter, brown sugar, and grated ginger. Mix until smooth.

● In another bowl, mix together the flour, bicarbonate of soda, cloves, nutmeg, and salt. Add to the molasses mixture together with the crystallized ginger. Mix well.

● Divide the mixture among the cups of the muffin tray. Bake for 20 minutes or until a skewer inserted into the centre of a muffin comes out clean.

● Serve the muffins warm with fresh pears, cut into wedges (or into thin slices for younger children).

Nutritional analysis per muffin with ½ pear	
calories	279
fat	10g (of which 5g is saturated)
protein	3g
carbohydrates	47g
fibre	1g
minerals	potassium
vitamins	A, B_1, B_2, B_3, B_6, folate
Food groups: carbs, dairy, fruits	

American pancakes

Makes 14 pancakes (4–5 servings)

200g (7oz) plain flour

60g (2¼oz) wholemeal flour

3 tablespoons caster sugar

2 teaspoons baking powder

½ teaspoon salt

2 eggs

360ml (12floz) skimmed milk

30g (1oz) butter, melted

150g (5oz) blueberries or other berries

Butter to grease the pan

● Sift the plain and wholemeal flours, sugar, baking powder, and salt into a large bowl. Tip in the bran from the sieve. Set aside.

● Break the eggs into a medium-sized bowl. Add the milk and melted butter, and whisk until everything is well mixed.

● Add the flour mixture to the egg mixture. Whisk until blended to make a batter. Gently fold in the blueberries.

● Heat some extra butter in a frying pan on moderate heat. It is hot enough when the butter starts to bubble.

● Use 6 tablespoons of batter for each pancake. Pour the measured batter into the pan; it will spread to make a pancake about 10cm (4 inches) in diameter. Cook three or four pancakes at a time, depending on the size of the pan. Cook until small bubbles appear on the top of the pancakes.

● Lift them with a spatula to see if they are light brown on the base. When they are, flip them over and cook for another few minutes until the pancakes are light brown on the other side.

● Serve hot, with syrup or fruit compote.

Nutritional analysis for 3 pancakes	
calories	305
fat	5g (of which 1g is saturated)
protein	11g
carbohydrates	52g
fibre	1g
minerals	calcium, potassium
vitamins	A, B_1, B_6, folate, C, D
Food groups: carbs, dairy, protein, fruits	

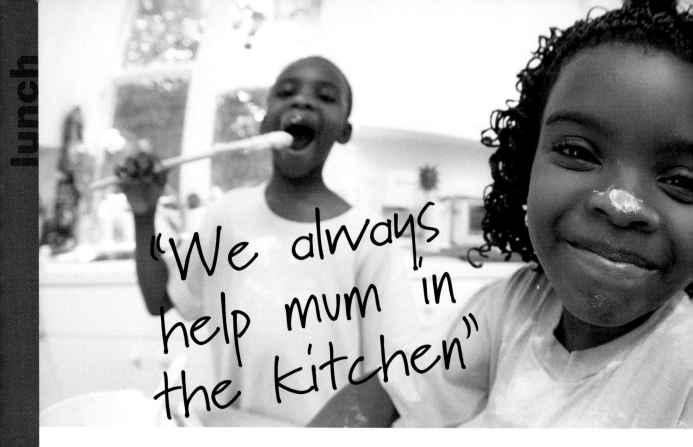

"We always help mum in the kitchen"

Take time for lunch

Tortellini kebabs

Makes 4 kebabs (4 servings)

170g (6oz) broccoli

12 medium to large frozen or dried
   cheese-filled tortellini

½ red pepper

½ cucumber, peeled

8 cherry tomatoes

Herb sauce

Juice of 1 lemon

4 teaspoons extra virgin olive oil

1–2 tablespoons chopped fresh herbs,
   such as basil, thyme, oregano,
   chives, mint, or coriander

Salt and pepper

● Trim the thick stalk from the broccoli and separate the florets. Drop them into a pan of boiling salted water and cook for 2 to 3 minutes or until just tender but still firm. Drain and rinse with cold water, then set aside.

● Cook the tortellini in boiling salted water until al dente (not too soft, still a little chewy). Drain and set aside to cool.

● Cut the red pepper and cucumber into 2.5-cm (1-inch) pieces. Arrange the pepper, cucumber, tortellini, broccoli, and tomatoes on four wooden skewers that are 10 to 15 cm (4 to 6 inches) long, alternating the ingredients. Lay the kebabs on a tray or large plate.

● To make the sauce, whisk together the ingredients, seasoning to taste with salt and pepper.

● Drizzle the sauce (or your child's favourite salad dressing) over the kebabs. Cover and chill for 1 hour, turning the kebabs occasionally. Serve chilled.

Nutritional analysis per kebab	
calories	134
fat	7g (of which 2g is saturated)
protein	3g
carbohydrates	15g
fibre	2.5g
minerals	calcium, potassium
vitamins	A, C, E
Food groups: carbs, dairy, vegetables	

Pleasing pitta pocket

Makes 1 pitta pocket (1 serving)

2 tablespoons hummus (traditional or
with roasted red pepper)

1 wholemeal pitta bread,
cut in half

30g (1oz) shredded lettuce

100g (3½oz) diced tomato

75g (2¾oz) diced cucumber

● Using a knife, spread 1 tablespoon hummus inside each pitta half, then add the lettuce, tomato, and cucumber.

● Serve as soon as possible, so the pitta bread doesn't soften.

Nutritional analysis per pocket	
calories	242
fat	5g (of which 0.4g is saturated)
protein	9g
carbohydrates	45g
fibre	6.5g
minerals	iron, potassium
vitamins	A, B_1, B_6, C

Food groups: carbs, protein, vegetables

Wild West wrap

Makes 2 servings

1 large flour tortilla

115g (4oz) cooked skinless, boneless
chicken breast, cut into strips or
small pieces

30g (1oz) Wensleydale or Cheddar
cheese, grated

30g (1oz) shredded lettuce

85g (3oz) diced tomato

1 tablespoon chunky salsa

● Lay the tortilla on a clean work surface. Arrange the chicken, cheese, lettuce, and tomato evenly down the centre of the tortilla. Spoon the salsa over the filling ingredients.

● Fold in the tortilla over one end of the filling, then roll up the tortilla tightly.

● Cut in half and serve.

Nutritional analysis per serving	
calories	217
fat	9g (of which 3g is saturated)
protein	23g
carbohydrates	13g
fibre	1g
minerals	potassium
vitamins	A, B_1, B_6, C

Food groups: carbs, dairy, protein, vegetables

Traditional quesadillas

Makes 4 quesadillas (4 servings)

Cooking spray

4 large flour tortillas

115g (4oz) Cheddar cheese, grated

85g (3oz) drained cooked or
canned black, red kidney,
or borlotti beans

85g (3oz) cooked frozen sweetcorn
kernels

Salsa, to serve

● Coat a frying pan with cooking spray and set it over medium heat. Place a tortilla in the pan.

● Sprinkle one-quarter of the cheese on half of the tortilla. Add 2 tablespoons beans and 2 tablespoons sweetcorn.

● Fold the other half of the tortilla over the filling and press down gently. Cook for 1 minute on each side until cheese melts.

● Remove the quesadilla from the pan and keep warm while you cook the rest.

● Serve the quesadillas cut into wedges, with salsa for dipping.

Nutritional analysis per quesadilla (without salsa)	
calories	299
fat	13g (of which 9g is saturated)
protein	14g
carbohydrates	33g
fibre	3.5g
minerals	calcium
vitamins	A, B_1, B_6

Food groups: carbs, dairy, protein, vegetables

Crunchy baked fish with lemon

Makes 4 servings

1 teaspoon butter

4 fresh white fish fillets, such as
    plaice, cod, halibut, or haddock,
    85g (3oz) each

Salt and pepper

Lemon juice

120ml (4floz) half-fat mayonnaise

100g (3½oz) fine dry breadcrumbs

2 teaspoons olive oil

Lemon wedges, to serve

● Preheat the oven to 180°C (350°F, gas mark 4). Use the butter to grease a baking tray.

● Arrange the fish fillets on the baking tray. Season the fish with salt and pepper. Drizzle a few drops of lemon juice over each fillet. Thinly spread the mayonnaise on top, then pat the breadcrumbs on to the mayonnaise. Finally, drizzle over the olive oil.

● Bake for 10 to 12 minutes, depending on the thickness of the fillets (test if the fish is cooked using the tip of a knife: the fish should flake easily).

● Serve hot, with lemon wedges.

Nutritional analysis per serving	
calories	305
fat 16g (of which 3g is saturated)	
protein	19g
carbohydrates	20g
fibre	0g
minerals	potassium
vitamins	B_{12}
Food groups: protein	

Home-made chicken soup

Makes 10 servings
(180ml/6floz each)

1 chicken, weighing 1.35–1.8kg
    (3–4lb)

Salt and pepper

1 teaspoon dried rosemary

2 bay leaves

2 teaspoons olive oil

1 onion, peeled and chopped

3 carrots, peeled and finely diced

3 celery sticks, finely diced

4 garlic cloves, peeled and crushed

1 large tomato, seeds removed and
    then diced

115g (4oz) fettuccine, broken into
    5-cm (2-inch) pieces

Juice of ¼ lemon

Grated nutmeg

● Rinse the chicken in cold water, then put it into a large pan. Cover with cold water and add salt and pepper, the rosemary, and bay leaves. Bring to the boil.

● Reduce the heat to moderate so the soup is simmering. Simmer for 40 minutes, skimming off the foam from the surface.

● Remove the chicken to a plate. Strain the broth and set aside.

● Wash the pan, then heat the olive oil in it on high heat. Add the onion, carrots, celery, garlic, and tomato. Cook, stirring, for 3 to 4 minutes.

● Add the chicken broth. Bring to the boil and simmer for 30 minutes.

● Meanwhile, take all the chicken meat from the bones. Discard the skin and cut the meat into small pieces.

● Add the pieces of chicken and the fettuccine pieces to the soup. Simmer for a further 10 to 15 minutes.

● Add the lemon juice and season with salt, pepper, and nutmeg to taste. Serve the soup hot.

● Home-made chicken soup can be kept in the refrigerator for up to four days; it also freezes well.

Nutritional analysis per serving	
calories	186
fat 6g (of which 2g is saturated)	
protein	18g
carbohydrates	13g
fibre	2.5g
minerals	potassium
vitamins	A, C
Food groups: protein, vegetables	

Turkey meatloaf sandwiches

Make this meatloaf the night before for sandwiches the next day. The recipe also can be doubled, to serve hot for dinner one night and lunch the next day.

Makes 8 sandwiches (8 servings)

Olive oil cooking spray

½ onion, peeled and finely chopped

1 carrot, peeled and finely diced

1 garlic clove, peeled and crushed

25g (scant 1oz) parsley, finely chopped

675g (1½lb) minced turkey

120ml (4floz) tomato passata

1 egg, lightly beaten

25g (scant 1oz) fresh breadcrumbs

Salt and pepper

120ml (4floz) tomato ketchup

16 slices of wholemeal bread,
   to serve

● Preheat the oven to 180°C (350°F, gas mark 4).

● Coat a frying pan with cooking spray and place over moderate heat. Add the onion, carrot, and garlic. Stir for 10 minutes until softened. Remove from the heat and leave the vegetables to cool.

● Add the parsley to the vegetables.

● In a large bowl, combine the minced turkey, vegetable mixture, passata, egg, and breadcrumbs. Season with some salt and pepper. Mix well together. Pack firmly into a greased loaf tin and top with the ketchup.

● Bake for 50 minutes. Remove from the oven and cover with aluminium foil. If serving the meatloaf hot, allow to stand for 10 minutes before cutting into eight slices. For sandwiches, leave the meatloaf to cool completely before slicing.

Nutritional analysis per sandwich	
calories	324
fat	11g (of which 3g is saturated)
protein	23g
carbohydrates	35g
fibre	5g
minerals	iron, potassium
vitamins	A, B_1, B_6, folate
Food groups: carbs, protein, vegetables	

Crispy courgette cake sandwiches

Makes 6 sandwiches (6 servings)

2 large courgettes, grated

1 teaspoon salt

115g (4oz) finely chopped onion

115g (4oz) finely diced peppers
   (half red, half green)

200g (7oz) well-drained, thawed
   frozen spinach

1 teaspoon chopped fresh basil

65g (2½oz) fresh breadcrumbs

1 egg

2 egg yolks

2 tablespoons half-fat mayonnaise

Salt and pepper

Paprika

Lemon juice

4 teaspoons olive oil

6 whole-grain bread rolls or baps,
   split open

● Place the grated courgettes in a sieve and add the salt. Toss together, then leave to drain for 20 minutes. With your hands, squeeze any remaining water out of the courgettes.

● In a large bowl, combine the courgettes, onion, peppers, spinach, and basil. Add the breadcrumbs.

● In a separate bowl, mix together the whole egg, egg yolks, and mayonnaise.

● Add the egg mixture to the courgette mixture and toss together. Season with salt, pepper, paprika, and lemon juice. Form the mixture into small cakes.

● Heat the olive oil in a frying pan on moderate heat. Cook the courgette cakes for 5 to 10 minutes on each side until crisp.

● Serve hot, in the whole-grain rolls.

Nutritional analysis per sandwich	
calories	275
fat	10g (of which 2g is saturated)
protein	10g
carbohydrates	39g
fibre	5g
minerals	iron, potassium
vitamins	A, folate, B_{12}, C, E, K
Food groups: carbs, vegetables	

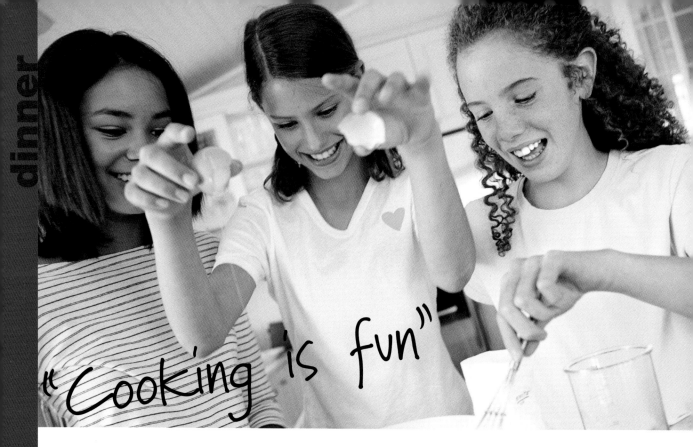

"Cooking is fun"

Sit down to dinner

Salad with pan-grilled chicken

Makes 4 servings

1 tablespoon chopped fresh rosemary
1 tablespoon chopped parsley
½ teaspoon garlic salt
4 chicken breasts without skin,
    about 170g (6oz) each
Cooking spray
125g (4½oz) chopped broccoli
65g (2½oz) chopped cauliflower
65g (2½oz) sliced carrots
65g (2½oz) chopped courgettes
65g (2½oz) sliced red onions
1 large tomato, diced
200g (7oz) mixed salad greens
2 tablespoons light dressing (optional)

● Sprinkle the rosemary, parsley, and garlic salt over the chicken breasts. Coat a ridged grill pan with cooking spray and heat it over medium-high heat. Pan-grill the chicken breasts until done, turning them over halfway through the cooking.

● Add the broccoli, cauliflower, carrots, courgettes, red onions, and tomato to the grill pan and cook for 2 minutes longer, stirring occasionally.

● Toss the salad greens with the dressing, if using, then pile on four plates. Top the greens with the chicken breasts and vegetables, and serve hot.

Nutritional analysis per serving (without dressing)	
calories	333
fat	7g (of which 2g is saturated)
protein	56g
carbohydrates	10g
fibre	3g
minerals	iron, potassium
vitamins	A, C, K
Food groups: protein, vegetables	

Mediterranean pasta soup

Makes 8 servings (240ml/8floz each)

2 teaspoons olive oil

85g (3oz) diced onion

360ml (12floz) water

480ml (16floz) chicken stock

½ teaspoon ground cumin

¼ teaspoon ground cinnamon

¼ teaspoon ground black pepper

1 can (about 400g/14oz) chickpeas, drained

1 can (about 400g/14oz) chopped tomatoes

85g (3oz) ditalini or other small pasta shapes

2 teaspoons chopped parsley

● Heat the olive oil in a large saucepan over moderate heat. Add the onion and sauté until lightly browned.

● Add the water, chicken stock, cumin, cinnamon, pepper, chickpeas, and canned tomatoes with their juice. Bring to the boil, then cover and reduce the heat. Simmer for 5 minutes.

● Add the pasta and stir, then cook for a further 10 minutes or until pasta is al dente (tender but still firm).

● Stir in the parsley. Serve hot.

Nutritional analysis per serving	
calories	119
fat 2g (of which 0.4g is saturated)	
protein	5g
carbohydrates	22g
fibre	2.5g
minerals	iron, potassium
vitamins	folate, C

Food groups: protein, vegetables

Cheesy quiche

A quiche is a great way to serve eggs to children. You can add whatever vegetables you have available, such as asparagus, broccoli, tomatoes, spinach, or mushrooms, or fresh herbs to the quiche filling. This recipe includes shortcrust pastry, but a ready-made pastry case works just as well.

Makes 8 servings

Shortcrust pastry

170g (6oz) plain flour

85g (3oz) butter

Pinch of salt

3 tablespoons cold water

Quiche filling

240ml (8floz) semi-skimmed milk

4 eggs

2 teaspoons plain flour

170g (6oz) mature Cheddar or Gruyère cheese, grated

Pinch of paprika

Salt and pepper

● First make the pastry. Sift the flour into a bowl and rub in the butter until the mixture resembles crumbs.

● Dissolve the salt in the water. Gradually add the water to the flour and butter mixture until it clumps together. Do not overwork or knead the pastry. Form it into a ball and wrap in greaseproof paper. Allow to rest for 30 minutes in the refrigerator.

● Preheat the oven to 180°C (350°F, gas mark 4). Put in a baking sheet to heat up. Roll out the pastry and use to line a 20-cm (8-inch) flan tin.

● To make the filling, combine all the ingredients, including any vegetables or herbs you'd like to add. Mix well and pour into the pastry case.

● Set the tin on the hot baking sheet. Bake for 45 to 55 minutes or until the pastry is golden brown and the filling is just set. Serve warm or cool. Cut into wedges for serving.

Nutritional analysis per serving	
calories	303
fat 20g (of which 11g is saturated)	
protein	12g
carbohydrates	18g
fibre	0.7g
minerals	calcium
vitamins	A, B_1, B_6, B_{12}, D, E

Food groups: carbs, dairy, protein

dinner

dinner

Pasta with fresh tomato sauce and basil

Makes 5 servings (150ml/¼ pint each)

450g (1lb) pasta

Freshly grated Parmesan cheese
(1 tablespoon each), to serve

Tomato sauce

3 tablespoons olive oil

2 garlic cloves, peeled and crushed

500g (1lb 2oz) ripe fresh tomatoes,
chopped, or 2 cans (about
400g/14oz each) chopped tomatoes

Salt and pepper

10g (scant ½oz) fresh basil leaves,
shredded

● To make the tomato sauce, heat the oil in a large saucepan over moderate heat. Add the garlic and cook for about 1 minute, stirring. Don't let it burn.

● Add the tomatoes and stir. Bring to the boil, then reduce the heat and simmer for about 10 minutes.

● Add salt and pepper to taste. Just before serving, stir the basil into the sauce and cook for 2 minutes.

● Cook the pasta in a large pan of boiling salted water until al dente (tender but still firm). Drain well. Pour the sauce over the pasta and toss together.

● Serve hot, with Parmesan cheese.

Nutritional analysis per serving	
calories	155
fat 3g (of which 0.1g is saturated)	
protein	5g
carbohydrates	25g
fibre	1g
minerals	–
vitamins	B$_1$, B$_6$, folate, C, E
Food groups: carbs, dairy, vegetables	

Vegetarian chilli

Makes 9 servings (240ml/8floz each)

2 tablespoons olive oil

1 onion, peeled and chopped

2 garlic cloves, peeled and finely
chopped

55g (2oz) chopped carrot

55g (2oz) chopped celery

55g (2oz) chopped red pepper

1 teaspoon ground cumin

1 teaspoon chilli powder, or to taste

Tabasco sauce or dried chilli flakes
to taste (optional)

2 cans (about 400g/14oz each)
chopped tomatoes

2 cans (about 400g/14oz each) red
kidney beans, drained and rinsed

150g (5oz) frozen sweetcorn kernels
(optional)

Salt and pepper

55g (2oz) Cheddar cheese, grated,
to serve

● Heat the oil in a heavy saucepan or flameproof casserole. Add the onion and garlic, and cook for 2 minutes. Add the carrot, celery, and red pepper, and cook until just tender, stirring occasionally.

● Stir in the cumin, chilli powder, and Tabasco sauce or chilli flakes, if using. Add the tomatoes with their juice and stir to mix. Bring to the boil, then reduce the heat and simmer for 15 to 20 minutes.

● Add the beans together with the sweetcorn, if using. Continue simmering until the beans and sweetcorn are heated through.

● Season to taste with salt and pepper. Serve hot, sprinkled with the cheese.

● If your child is interested in a vegetarian diet, this is a great dish to try. Serve it over noodles or bulgur wheat.

Nutritional analysis per serving (without sweetcorn)	
calories	157
fat 4g (of which 1g is saturated)	
protein	7g
carbohydrates	24g
fibre	5g
minerals	potassium
vitamins	A, C, E
Food groups: protein, vegetables	

Traditional meat sauce for pasta or gnocchi

This sauce tastes better if it is made in a big batch. It freezes well and also can be kept in the refrigerator for three to five days. It is great on spaghetti or any other kind of pasta, or on gnocchi.

**Makes 12 servings
(180ml/6floz each)**
900g (2lb) minced very lean beef
2 onions, peeled and finely
    chopped
6 carrots, peeled and diced
1 celeriac, peeled and diced,
    or 3 celery sticks, diced
75g (2¾oz) mushrooms, sliced
4 large tomatoes, diced
3 garlic cloves, peeled and crushed
115g (4oz) tomato paste
1 teaspoon each dried oregano, dried
    thyme, dried basil, dried rosemary,
    and paprika

2 bay leaves
1.5 litres (2½ pints) vegetable or beef
    stock
750ml (1¼ pints) water
Salt and pepper
Pasta or gnocchi, to serve

● Put the minced beef into a large saucepan and brown over moderate heat, stirring to break up lumps.
● Add the onions, carrots, celeriac or celery, mushrooms, tomatoes, and garlic. Stir in the tomato paste, dried herbs, paprika, and bay leaves. Cook for a further 10 minutes, stirring frequently.
● Add the stock and water, and bring to the boil. Reduce the heat, cover, and simmer gently for 2 to 3 hours.
● Season to taste with salt and pepper.
● Toss the sauce with pasta or gnocchi that has been cooked and drained.

Nutritional analysis per serving (without pasta or gnocchi)

calories	257
fat	14g (of which 6g is saturated)
protein	21g
carbohydrates	11g
fibre	3g
minerals	iron, potassium
vitamins	A, B$_{12}$, C

Food groups: protein, vegetables

Salmon burgers

Makes 5 burgers (5 servings)
2 cans (about 180g/6½oz each) salmon,
    drained
1 egg, lightly beaten
55g (2oz) finely chopped green
    or red pepper
30g (1oz) fresh wholemeal breadcrumbs
1 teaspoon grated lemon zest
1 teaspoon lemon juice
½ teaspoon dried rosemary, crushed
Pinch each of salt and pepper
1 teaspoon olive oil

● Combine all the ingredients, except the olive oil, in a bowl and mix well. Form into five burgers.
● Heat the olive oil in a non-stick frying pan on moderate heat. Add the burgers and fry for 4 minutes on each side or until lightly browned.
● Serve the salmon burgers hot, in whole-grain baps or with a favourite vegetable or salad.

Nutritional analysis per burger (without bap)

calories	211
fat	11g (of which 1g is saturated)
protein	21g
carbohydrates	8g
fibre	0g
minerals	–
vitamins	C

Food groups: protein

Snacks and smoothies

Trail mix

Makes 7 servings (120ml/4floz each)

75g (2¾oz) sultanas

75g (2¾oz) dried cranberries

55g (2oz) dried apricots

40g (1½oz) unsalted peanuts

40g (1½oz) blanched, halved almonds

40g (1½oz) chocolate chips (optional)

40g (1½oz) sunflower seeds

40g (1½oz) crunchy oat cereal or
    granola

● Combine all the ingredients in a container with a lid or in a bag. Trail Mix will keep, sealed, for about three weeks in a cool, dry place.

Nutritional analysis per serving (without chocolate chips)	
calories	208
fat 8g (of which 6g is saturated)	
protein	6g
carbohydrates	36g
fibre	7g
minerals	potassium, zinc
vitamins	folate, B_{12}, E
Food groups: carbs, protein	

Healthy bean salsa

Makes 10 servings (120ml/4floz each)

1 onion, peeled and finely chopped

4 tablespoons chopped fresh coriander

1 can (about 425g/15oz) black beans,
    drained and rinsed

1 can (about 310g/10½oz) sweetcorn
    kernels, drained

1 can (about 400g/14oz) chopped
    tomatoes

1 can (about 120g/4¼oz) diced
    chillies, drained

Juice of ½ lime

● Combine all the ingredients and serve with tortilla chips.

Nutritional analysis per serving	
calories	77
fat .4g (of which 0.1g is saturated)	
protein	3g
carbohydrates	16g
fibre	4g
minerals	potassium
vitamins	folate
Food groups: protein, vegetables	

Apple bars

Makes about 24 bars (1 serving each)

115g (4oz) soft butter

200g (7oz) caster sugar

1 egg, beaten

200g (7oz) plain flour

½ teaspoon bicarbonate of soda

½ teaspoon grated nutmeg

225g (8oz) diced apples

Topping

55g (2oz) soft light brown sugar

65g (2½oz) chopped walnuts

½ teaspoon grated nutmeg

½ teaspoon ground cinnamon

● Preheat the oven to 180°C (350°F, gas mark 4).

● Cream the butter and sugar together. Add the egg and mix well.

● In another bowl, stir together the flour, bicarbonate of soda, and nutmeg. Add to the creamed mixture and blend well. Mix in the apples. Spread the mixture in a greased 30 x 20cm (12 x 8 inch) tin.

● Combine the ingredients for the topping and scatter evenly over the mixture.

● Bake for 30 minutes. Cool in the tin before cutting into bars for serving.

Nutritional analysis per bar	
calories	130
fat 6g (of which 3g is saturated)	
protein	1g
carbohydrates	19g
fibre	1g
minerals	zinc
vitamins	E
Food groups: carbs, fruit	

Strawberry-banana smoothie

Makes 2 servings
(300ml/½ pint each)

240ml (8floz) semi-skimmed milk

120ml (4floz) silken tofu

75g (2¾oz) sliced bananas

125g (4½oz) sliced fresh or frozen
   unsweetened strawberries

Coarsely crushed ice

● Put all the ingredients in a blender or food processor and blend until smooth and frothy. Serve immediately.

● Instead of semi-skimmed milk, you can use skimmed milk or substitute soya or rice milk. Note, though, that soya milk contains considerably less calcium than cow's milk and rice milk has less protein.

Nutritional analysis per serving	
calories	136
fat	5g (of which 1g is saturated)
protein	10g
carbohydrates	16g
fibre	2.5g
minerals	calcium, potassium
vitamins	B$_{12}$, C, D
Food groups: dairy, protein, fruits	

Fruit-nutty smoothie

Makes 3 servings
(about 360ml/12floz each)

240ml (8floz) low-fat plain yogurt

240ml (8floz) semi-skimmed milk

400g (14oz) sliced fresh or frozen
   unsweetened strawberries

1 fresh peach, peeled and sliced, or
   125g (4½oz) frozen unsweetened
   peach slices

2 teaspoons pure vanilla extract

To garnish

2 tablespoons chopped walnuts

Whole strawberries

● Put all the ingredients (except the garnish) in a blender or food processor and blend until smooth and frothy.

● Pour into glasses and garnish, then serve.

Nutritional analysis per serving	
calories	160
fat	5.5g (of which 1g is saturated)
protein	7g
carbohydrates	20g
fibre	1.5g
minerals	calcium, potassium
vitamins	A, B$_{12}$, C, D
Food groups: dairy, protein, fruits	

Berry good smoothie

Makes 2 servings
(about 360ml/12floz each)

240ml (8floz) semi-skimmed milk

120ml (4floz) silken tofu

55g (2oz) fresh or frozen unsweetened
   blueberries

40g (1½oz) fresh or frozen unsweetened
   raspberries

85g (3oz) sliced fresh or frozen
   unsweetened strawberries

Coarsely crushed ice

● Put all the ingredients in a blender or food processor and blend until smooth and frothy. Serve immediately.

Nutritional analysis per serving	
calories	129
fat	5g (of which 1g is saturated)
protein	9.5g
carbohydrates	15g
fibre	2.5g
minerals	calcium, potassium
vitamins	B$_{12}$, C, D
Food groups: dairy, protein, fruits	

smoothies

Recommended resources

Food and nutrition

British Dietetic Association
5th floor, Charles House
148/9 Great Charles Street, Queensway
Birmingham B3 3HT
www.bda.uk.com

British Nutrition Foundation
High Holborn House
52–54 High Holborn,
London WC1V 6RQ
www.nutrition.org.uk

European Food Information Council (EUFIC)
19 rue Guimard
1040 Brussels, Belgium
www.eufic.org/gb/home/home.htm

Food Standards Agency
England: Aviation House
125 Kingsway
London WC2B 6NH
Scotland: St Magnus House, 6th floor
25 Guild Street
Aberdeen AB11 6NJ
Wales: 11th floor, Southgate House
Wood Street,
Cardiff CF10 1EW
www.foodstandards.gov.uk

KidsHealth
This website offers doctor-approved health information for children and teenagers, as well as parents. The topics covered include food, fitness, and weight concerns.
www.kidshealth.org

La Leche League
This international organization provides information, support, and advocacy for breastfeeding mothers.
www.lalecheleague.org

The Vegetarian Society
Parkdale
Dunham Road
Altrincham, Cheshire WA14 4QG
www.vegsoc.org

Weight Concern
Brook House
2–16 Torrington Place
London WC1E 7HN
www.weightconcern.com

Physical activity and sport

Department for Culture, Media and Sport
2–4 Cockspur Street
London SW1Y 5DH
www.culture.gov.uk

Sports Council for Northern Ireland
House of Sport
Upper Malone Road
Belfast BT9 5LA
www.sportni.net

Sports Council for Wales
Sophia Gardens
Cardiff CF11 9SW
www.sports-council-wales.co.uk

Sport England
3rd floor, Victoria House
Bloomsbury Square,
London WC1B 4SE
www.sportengland.org

Sport Scotland
Caledonia House
South Gyle
Edinburgh EH12 9DQ
www.sportscotland.org.uk

UK Sport

40 Bernard Street
London WC1N 1ST
www.uksport.gov.uk

Youth Sport Trust

Sir John Beckwith Centre for Sport
Loughborough University
Loughborough, Leicestershire LE11 3TU
www.youthsporttrust.org

Websites for various sports and activities

archery www.gnas.org
baseball www.baseballsoftballuk.com
basketball www.fibaeurope.com
baton twirling www.nbta.org.uk
climbing and mountaineering www.thebmc.co.uk
croquet www.croquet.org.uk
curling www.britishcurlingassociation.org.uk
fencing www.britishfencing.com
footbag www.footbagger.co.uk
football www.thefa.com
geocaching www.geocaching.com
golf www.englishgolfunion.com
gymnastics www.british-gymnastics.org
ice skating www.iceskating.org.uk
juggling www.juggling.org
laser tag www.lasertag.org
orienteering www.britishorienteering.org.uk
paintball www.paintball.co.uk
rowing www.ara-rowing.org
rugby www.rfu.com
taekwondo www.sporttaekwondouk.staffs.org
volleyball www.volleyballengland.org

Children with special needs

Anaphylaxis Campaign

PO Box 275
Farnborough, Hampshire GU14 6SX
Helpline: 01252 542 029
www.anaphylaxis.org.uk

Diabetes UK

10 Parkway, London NW1 7AA
Careline: 020 7424 1030
www.diabetes.org.uk

Eating Disorders Association

103 Prince of Wales Road, Norwich NR1 1DW
Youth line: 0845 634 7650
www.edauk.com

National Asthma Campaign

Providence House, Providence Place, London N1 0NT
Helpline: 08457 010 203
www.asthma.org.uk

British Paralympic Association

Norwich Union Building, 9th floor
69 Park Lane
Croydon, Surrey CR9 1BG
www.paralympics.org.uk

British Wheelchair Sports Foundation

Stoke Mandeville Stadium, Guttmann Road,
Stoke Mandeville, Buckinghamshire HP21 9PP
www.bwsf.org.uk

Royal Association for Disability and Rehabilitation (RADAR)

12 City Forum, 250 City Road
London EC1V 8AF
www.radar.org.uk

Special Olympics Great Britain

National Development Office,
18 Grosvenor Gardens,
London SW1W 0DH
www.specialolympicsgb.org

Holiday Care Service

7th floor, Sunley House
Croydon, Surrey CR0 2AP
www.holidaycare.org.uk

Index

A

activity log 60, 62
activity menu 60
adolescents 148–69
  dieting 162–3
  fitness 54, 164–9
  jobs 169
  nutrition 152–63
advertisements, for food 29,
    115, 133
aerobic exercise 56
alcohol 155
allergies
  asthma 178–9
  food allergies 78, 79,
    174–5
American pancakes 191
amino acids 35
anaphylaxis 175
anorexia nervosa 147, 163
apple bars 200
archery 142
arm curl exercise 58
ascorbic acid 39
asthma 178–9
athletic children 136–7, 145,
    182–5
attention deficit hyperactivity
    disorder (ADHD) 120,
    179

B

babies 68–91
  activity 54, 84–91
  feeding 70–1, 72–83
  night feeds 83
  overweight 71
  physical development 71,
    85
  play 88, 89, 91
  safety 86, 90

  self-feeding 82–3
  winding 76
baby carriers 87
baby food 80
Balance of Good Health
    40–1
bananas, strawberry-banana
    smoothie 201
basketball 65, 137
baton twirling 142
beans
  healthy bean salsa 200
  vegetarian chilli 198
beef, traditional meat sauce
    for pasta or gnocchi 199
berry good smoothie 201
binge eating 147, 163
blood sugar levels
  diabetes 151, 176, 177
  glycaemic index 34
Body Mass Index (BMI)
    18–19, 147
bones, calcium and 157
bottlefeeding 72, 76–7
  benefits of 74
  feeding schedule 73
  how much to feed 77
  stopping 100
  types of formula 77
  winding baby 76
bowel movements, babies 79
breakfast
  adolescents 153–4, 156,
    161
  pre-school children 114
  recipes 190–1
  school-age children 130,
    133
  toddlers 97
breastfeeding 72, 74–6
  benefits of 74
  feeding schedule 73

  problems 74
  stopping 100
  winding baby 76
breathing problems
  asthma 178–9
  overweight children 22
bulimia nervosa 147, 163
burgers, salmon 199

C

caffeine 116–17, 183
calcium 38, 39
  adolescent diet 156–7
  athletic children 183
  food labels 48
  pre-school children's diet
    112
  school-age children's diet
    132
  toddlers' diet 96
  vegetarian diet 159
calf stretch exercise 57
calories 33
  adolescent diet 153, 156
  athletic children 183
  babies' needs 70
  in cola 116
  food labels 48
  pre-school children's diet
    112
  school-age children's diet
    127, 132
  toddlers' diet 96
camps
  summer camps 141, 181
  weight-loss camps 147
canned food 47
carbohydrates 34
  adolescent diet 153
  athletic children 183
  carbohydrate foods 40, 41
  and diabetes 176

  food labels 48
  school-age children's diet
    127
carbohydrate foods
  Balance of Good Health
    40–1
  fibre content 34–5
  toddlers' diet 95
cereal
  breakfast cereal 127, 154
  hearty Swiss muesli 190
  infant cereal 78–9
cheese
  cheesy quiche 197
  traditional quesadillas 193
chicken
  home-made chicken soup
    194
  salad with pan-grilled
    chicken 196
  Wild West wrap 193
childcare 86, 107
chilli, vegetarian 198
choking 83
cholesterol 36
  fibre and 34
  food labels 48
cola 15, 116
computer games 29, 62, 121
conflict at mealtimes 101–2
contracts, fitness 60, 167
convenience food 14, 42, 47
cooking 188–9
  involving children 45, 117,
    131
cooling-down exercises 64
coordination, baby's 88
courgette cake sandwiches,
    crispy 195
crawling 91
cricket 65, 137
croquet 142

cups, introducing 83, 100
curl-ups exercise 59, 63
curling 142
cycling 137

D

daily nutritional requirements
32, 33, 48
dairy foods
adolescent diet 157
Balance of Good Health
40–1
lactose intolerance 175
toddlers' diet 95
see also cheese; milk;
yogurt
dancing 137
dehydration 67, 116, 182–3
diabetes 21, 176–7
carbohydrates and 34
exercise and 177
hypoglycaemia 177
nutrition needs 176
overweight children and
151
screening for 151
dieting 147, 162–3
dietitians 23, 173
disabled children 180–1
doctors 23, 173
drinks
calorie content 15
cola 15, 116
and exercise 67
pre-school children
116–17
thirst 67, 116–17
water 36, 67, 116, 182–3

E

eating disorders 147, 163
eating habits 12–13, 113
eating out 27
emotions, using food to
relieve 114

endurance, physical fitness
56
energy, calories 33
equipment, sports 65, 66,
139
evening meal (dinner, tea)
adolescents 156, 161
pre-school children 114
recipes 196–9
school-age children 130,
133
toddlers 97
exercise see fitness
eye appeal
colourful food 33
pre-school children's diet
113

F

family approach, lifestyle
changes 24–9
family meals 15
adolescents 152, 155
conflict 101–2
school-age children 133
fast food
adolescent diet 162
eating out 27
limiting 42
portion sizes 14
television advertisements
115, 133
fat, Body Mass Index (BMI)
18–19, 147
fats, dietary 35–6
adolescent diet 153
athletic children 183
food labels 48
low-fat diets 43
school-age children's diet
127
female athlete triad 185
fencing 137
fibre 34–5
adolescent diet 153

pre-school children's diet
112
school-age children's diet
127
toddlers' diet 96
finger foods 82, 83, 98
fish
crunchy baked fish with
lemon 194
and vegetarian diet 159
fitness 50–67
activity for babies 84–91
adolescents 164–9
and asthma 178–9
athletic children 182
benefits of exercise 52–3,
54
and diabetes 177
disabled children 180–1
exercise drinks 67
how much exercise? 54
lifestyle changes 28–9
measuring 62–3
motivation 55, 60–1, 138,
166–7
pre-school children
118–21
safety 64–6
school-age children 125,
136–45
sedentary lifestyle 15,
28–9
toddlers 104–7
fitness contracts 60, 167
flexibility 56, 57
folate 39
food allergies 78, 79, 174–5
food logs 42–3
food poisoning 49
food sensitivities 175
football 65, 137
safety gear 65
free play 55
pre-school children
118–19

school-age children 138,
145
toddlers 106
frozen food 47
fruit
Balance of Good Health
40–1
fibre content 34–5
five-a-day servings 43
frozen and canned food 47
hearty Swiss muesli 190
introducing solid foods 73,
79
shopping 46–8
storing 47
toddlers' diet 95
see also juice
fruit-nutty smoothie 201
fussy eaters 44–5, 95

G

gardening, for children 111
geocaching 165
gingerbread muffins 191
giving up sports 144
glycaemic index (GI) 34
gnocchi, traditional meat
sauce for 199
golf 137, 142
"grazing" 115
growth
adolescents 150–1, 156
babies 77
growth charts 16–17
pre-school children 112
puberty 146–7
school-age children 132
toddlers 95
gymnastics 15, 137, 141

H

health problems 21–2,
171–85
heart disease 21, 34, 155
heat-related illnesses 67, 182

height
    Body Mass Index (BMI)
        18–19, 147
    see also growth charts
helmets 66
hockey 65, 137
hunger
    babies 70–1, 77
    pre-school children 111,
        114, 115
    recognizing cues 12, 26
hydrogenated oils 36
hygiene, food preparation 49
hyperactivity 120, 179
hypoglycaemia 177

I

immunologists 173
infants see babies
injuries 65, 67
    athletic children 184
insulin
    carbohydrates and 34
    diabetes 21, 151, 176
iron 38, 39
    adolescent diet 156, 157
    athletic children 183
    food labels 48
    in formula milk 76
    pre-school children's diet
        112
    toddlers' diet 96, 97
    vegetarian diet 159

J

jobs, adolescents 169
juice
    for babies 80
    calorie content 15, 116

K

kebabs, tortellini 192
kitchen safety 49
knee pain, overweight
    children 22

L

labels, food 48, 132, 133
lacrosse, safety gear 65
lactose intolerance 76, 132,
    175
language development 111
leg lift exercise 59
low-fat diets 43
lunches
    adolescents 156, 161
    packed lunches 128, 129
    pre-school children 114
    recipes 192–5
    school-age children 130,
        133
    school meals 126, 128–9
    toddlers 97

M

martial arts 137
meat
    introducing solid foods 73
    meat sauce for pasta or
        gnocchi 199
    vegetarian alternatives 159
Mediterranean pasta soup
    197
menstruation
    anorexia and 163
    overweight girls 22
    starting 150, 156
menu planning 188
    adolescents 156, 161
    pre-school children 114
    school-age children 130,
        133
    toddlers 97
milk
    in adolescent diet 157
    alternative sources of
        calcium 132
    bottlefeeding 72, 73,
        76–7, 100
    breastfeeding 74–6

introducing cups 83, 100
    for pre-school children 116
    smoothies 201
    in toddlers' diet 95, 96–7
minerals 38–9
    food labels 48
    fortified breakfast cereals
        127
    supplements 38
    vegetarian diet 159
monounsaturated fats 36
motivation, for exercise 60–1
    adolescents 166–7
    overweight children 55
    school-age children 138
muffins, gingerbread with
    fresh pears 191

N

new foods
    fussy eaters 44–5, 95
    introducing solids 72, 73,
        78–81
    pre-school children's diet
        113
    toddlers' diet 98
niacin 39
night feeds, babies 83
non-athletic children 61,
    144–5
nutrition 32–49
    adolescents 152–63
    athletic children 183
    babies 72–83
    pre-school children 112–17
    school-age children 124,
        126–35
    toddlers 95–103

O

occupational therapists 173
omega-3 fatty acids 36
orange juice 116
orthopaedic surgeons 173
osteoporosis 157

outings 29
overhead stretch exercise 57
overweight children 20–3
    babies 71
    Body Mass Index (BMI) 18
    emotional problems 21
    exercise 55
    health problems 21–2,
        151
    lifestyle changes 23–9

P

packed lunches 128, 129
pancakes, American 191
pasta
    introducing solid foods 73
    Mediterranean pasta soup
        197
    tortellini kebabs 192
    traditional meat sauce for
        pasta 199
    with fresh tomato sauce
        and basil 198
peanut allergy 174
pears, gingerbread muffins
    with 191
pedometers 61
periods see menstruation
personality
    babies 80–1
    and fitness 61
physical education classes 15,
    138–9, 141
physical fitness see fitness
physiotherapists 173
picnics 117
pitta pocket, pleasing 193
pizzas 131
play 55
    babies 88, 89, 91
    pre-school children 118–19
    school-age children 138,
        145
    toddlers 106
playgrounds, safety 121

polyunsaturated fats 36

portion sizes 41

    fast food 14

    toddlers 103

potassium 39

potatoes, introducing solid
    foods 73

pre-school children 108–21

    computers 121

    feeding 112–17

    fitness 54, 118–21

    individuality 110–11

    physical development 119

    safety 121

    thirst 116–17

press-ups exercise 59, 63

pretend play 119

protein 35

    adolescent diet 153

    athletic children 183

    Balance of Good Health
        40–1

    food labels 48

    pre-school children's diet
        112

    school-age children's diet
        127

    toddlers' diet 95, 96

    vegetarian diet 159

puberty 146–7, 150

    eating disorders 147

    nutrition and 156

    signs of 147

    weight gain 18, 147

pull out exercise 58

purées, baby food 80

Q

quesadillas, traditional 193

quiche, cheesy 197

R

reading 111

regurgitating, babies 77

resistance band exercises 58

restaurants 27, 162

retinol 39

rewards, food as 45, 102

riboflavin 39

rice, introducing solid foods
    73

road safety 66, 121

role models, parents as 13,
    15, 43, 151

rollerblading 137

    safety gear 65

rowing exercise 58

rugby 137

    safety gear 65

running 137

S

safety

    babies 86, 90

    exercise programmes
        64–5

    in kitchen 49

    packed lunches 128

    pre-school children 121

    road safety 66, 121

    toddlers 106–7

    walking to school 145

    water 66

salmon burgers 199

salsa, healthy bean 200

salt 38

sandwiches 195

saturated fat 36

school-age children 122–47

    cooking with 131

    fitness 54, 125, 136–45

    nutrition 124, 126–35

    puberty 146–7

    snacks 130, 131, 133, 134

schools

    meals 126, 128–9

    preparing children for 120

    vending machines 128,
        154

scooters 65

seat drop exercise 59

sedentary lifestyle 15, 28–9,
    62

serving sizes 41, 48

shoes, for toddlers 105

shopping 26, 46–8

shuttle run 63

sit and reach test 63

sit and twist exercise 57

sit-ups exercise 63

sitting up, babies 89

skateboarding, safety gear 65

skating 137

sleep problems 22

slings, baby 87

smoking 155, 157

smoothies 201

snacks

    adolescent diet 154, 156,
        161, 162

    athletic children 183

    limiting 27, 42

    pre-school children 114,
        115

    recipes 200

    school-age children 130,
        131, 133, 134

    television advertising 29

    toddlers 97, 100

sodium 38, 48

solid foods, introducing 72,
    73, 78–81

soups

    home-made chicken soup
        194

    Mediterranean pasta soup
        197

    vegetable soup for baby 83

special needs, children with
    180–1

sport

    and ADHD 179

    adolescents 165

    and asthma 179

    athletic children 182–5

disabled children 181

    equipment 65, 66, 139

    giving up 144

    organized sports 55

    pre-school children 121

    school-age children 125,
        137, 139–40, 142–3,
        145

sports drinks 183

sports medicine doctors 173

sports supplements 185

standing up, babies 89

steroids 184, 185

storing food 47, 49

strawberries

    fruit-nutty smoothie 201

    strawberry-banana
        smoothie 201

strength, physical fitness 56,
    58–9

stretching exercises 57

Sudden Infant Death
    Syndrome (SIDS) 87

sugar 34

summer camps 141, 181

sunblock 66

supplements

    sports supplements 185

    vitamins and minerals 26,
        38

surgeons, orthopaedic 173

sweets

    conflicts over 102

    limiting 27

    as a reward 12

swimming 66, 137

T

tantrums, toddlers 101

team sports 139–40, 142–3,
    145

teenagers see adolescents

television

    advertisements 29, 115,
        133

eating in front of 15

limiting 29, 62, 106

temperament see personality

tennis 137

thiamin 39

thigh stretch exercise 57

thirst 67, 116–17

tiredness 22

toddlers 92–107

activity 54, 104–7

feeding 95–103

food preferences 98–100

fussy eaters 95

physical development 105

safety 106–7

self-feeding 101–2

tooth care 100

tomatoes, pasta with fresh

tomato sauce 198

tooth care, toddlers 100

tortellini kebabs 192

trail mix 200

trampolines 65

trans fats 36

treats 42, 45

turkey meatloaf sandwiches

195

U

university, going to 161

unsaturated fats 36

V

vegan diet 159

vegetables

Balance of Good Health

40–1

fibre content 34–5

five-a-day servings 43

frozen and canned food

47

introducing solid foods 73,

79

shopping 46–8

storing 47

toddlers' diet 95

vegetarian chilli 198

vegetarian diet 35, 38, 159

vending machines, at school

128, 154

videos 29, 107

vitamins 26, 38–9, 48

fortified breakfast cereals

127

supplements 26, 38

vegetarian diet 159

vomiting, bulimia 147, 163

W

walking

babies' development 90

pre-school children 120

to school 145

toddlers 105

warming-up exercises 64

water 36, 67, 116, 182–3

safety 66

weight, Body Mass Index

(BMI) 18–19, 147

weight gain

athletic children 185

babies 71

growth charts 16–17

in puberty 18, 147

weight loss, athletic children

184–5

weight-loss camps 147

weight training 58

Wild West wrap 193

winding babies 76

work, adolescents 169

Y

yogurt, fruit-nutty smoothie

201

Z

zinc 39

vegetarian diet 159

Acknowledgments

KidsHealth

We would like to thank the following organizations for their important work in childhood fitness and nutrition:
American Academy of Pediatrics; American Dietetic Association; American Heart Association; American Medical Association Centers for Disease Control and Prevention; US Department of Health and Human Services; National Association for Sport and Physical Education; National Institutes of Health; President's Council on Physical Fitness and Sports; US Department of Agriculture; US Surgeon General's Office; YMCA.
We also acknowledge the wonderful work of the following people: Erica Blacksburg; Allison Brinkley, RD; Beth Dowshen; Debra Duby; Randy B. Garber; Cathy Ginther; Mary Lou Jay; Marissa Lippert; D'Arcy Lyness, PhD; James M. Poole, MD; Eric Small, MD; Shaynee Snider; Amy Sutton; Eve Tahmincioglu; Laura Winchester.

Dorling Kindersley

We would like to thank Hilary Bird for the index; Salima Hirani and Kathryn Wilkinson for editorial help; Isabel de Cordova, Sara Kimmins, Iona Hoyle, and Cath McKenzie for design help.

Photography Janeanne Gilchrist, Unit Photographic.

Growth Charts are based on information and charts supplied by the Child Growth Foundation, which are subject to copyright. Originals of the growth charts can be purchased from Harlow Printing, Maxwell Street, South Shields NE33 4PU.

Picture Credits

Allsport Concepts (Getty) 65

Botanica (Getty) 94

Foodpix (Getty) 25tr, 39, 73, 79, 101, 116, 154, 158

Image Bank (Getty) 2tl, 22, 25br, 30, 32, 45, 54, 55, 61, 70, 74, 99, 100, 102, 104, 134, 135, 143, 144, 155, 160, 164, 174, 177, 178, 179, 180, 182, 185

Photographers Choice (Getty) 36

Royalty Free Images (Getty) 16, 82, 126, 139, 170

Stone (Getty) 7bl, 8, 13, 20, 21, 40, 56, 71, 72, 81, 84, 86, 88, 90, 91, 107, 111, 115, 117, 119, 131, 142, 146, 159, 163, 174, 175, 176, 181, 186

Taxi (Getty) 2br, 6bl, 7br, 12, 17, 24, 27, 35, 43, 44, 50, 53, 60, 63, 68, 78, 85, 87, 89, 92, 96, 98, 105t, 105b, 106, 108, 110, 112, 118, 127, 132, 137, 140, 145, 151, 152, 161, 162, 165, 166, 168, 169, 188, 190, 192, 196

All other images © Dorling Kindersley. For further information see www.dkimages.com